D1491054

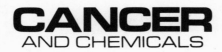

CANCER
AND CHEMICALS

THOMAS H. CORBETT, M.D.

CANCER
AND CHEMICALS

Nelson - Hall / Chicago

Library of Congress Cataloging in Publication Data

Corbett, Thomas H
  Cancer and chemicals.

  Includes index.
  1. Carcinogens.   2. Environmentally induced diseases.
3. Cancer.   I. Title.
RC268.6.C67   616.9'94'071   76-54270
ISBN 0-88229-305-2 (Cloth)
ISBN 0-88229-465-2 (Paper)

Manufactured in the United States of America

To my father and my mother:

Thomas Cyril Corbett
1895–1976

Dorothy Marie Huhmann Corbett

Contents

Introduction

Past civilizations have been decimated by plagues of bacterial and viral diseases, which we have learned to prevent through medical and scientific research. It is unlikely that plagues of transmittable diseases will occur in our civilization. However, Mother Nature, in her infinite wisdom, is providing us with a new category of diseases to replace the ones we have prevented. Ironically, these new diseases are caused by the very by-products of our ability to prevent the old ones. These by-products are the pollutants of our highly industrialized and technological society. Dr. Irving J. Selikoff of New York's Mount Sinai School of Medicine has called environmental disease "the disease of the century."

This book discusses environmental disease and describes the chemicals that are polluting our environment: what they are, where they are, how they got there, and most important, what effects they have on our health and well-being. The final chapter explains how each of us individually can minimize the risk.

This book should show the reader that the most devastating

of the environmental diseases is cancer. And related to cancer are environmentally produced mutations and birth defects. Statistics now show that the United States has one of the world's highest incidences of cancer associated with environmental pollution. The increase in cancer rates observed today is the result of exposure twenty years ago to cancer-producing chemicals. Considering the thousands of untested new chemicals introduced into the environment each year, the incidence of cancer should skyrocket to epidemic proportions by the beginning of the twenty-first century.

The best solution to the problem of environmental disease is prevention. Some two million chemical compounds—many of them man-made—are now known to exist. It is estimated that 25,000 new chemicals are developed each year, and of this total about 10,000 have significant commercial applications. Although most of these chemicals are not dangerous, the few that are could decimate our population if used indiscriminately. The dangerous chemicals must be screened and prohibited before they are used in products or manufacturing processes.

1
Too Many People, Too Many Machines

And one is a teacher and one a beginner
Just wanting to be there and wanting to know
And together they're trying to tell us a story
That should have been listened to long, long ago
How the life in the mountains is living in danger
From too many people, too many machines
And the time is upon us, today is forever
Tomorrow is just one of yesterday's dreams
John Denver*

We live in the greatest technological age that man has ever known. We have conquered diseases that used to kill millions of people before maturity, robbing them of a full life span. We have made survival infinitely easier and allowed man leisure time for learning, for enjoyment, and for fulfillment of his desires and dreams.

Rocky Mountain Suite (Cold Nights in Canada) by John Denver. © Copyright 1973 Cherry Lane Music Co. Used by permission. All rights reserved.

1

We have sent man beyond our own planet to the moon, and we have explored even farther with our machines. Pioneer 10 has revealed that the planet Jupiter is a huge mass of hydrogen gas with a liquid hydrogen center hotter than the sun. Pioneer 11 has confirmed these findings and is speeding on to explore Saturn. Data from the space program indicate that other planets in our solar system are also inhospitable to life.

These findings undermine our previous conceptions of the planets, including thoughts of colonizing Venus and Mars. We can no longer entertain images of races of giants inhabiting Jupiter or supercivilizations existing elsewhere in our solar system. Perhaps billions of years ago other planets in our solar system may have been capable of supporting life and perhaps billions of years in the future some other planets will have a life capability. But right now we are here, alone, and there is no place else for us to go. If we destroy our planet's delicate balance of nature and its ability to sustain life, we shall also destroy ourselves.

We as human beings are made of chemicals, constantly reacting and interacting to sustain the condition we call life. Life depends on exquisitely balanced processes, and it takes very little to interfere with or destroy the reactions that sustain it. Common examples of such interference are poisoning and disease.

The delicate balance of conditions allowing us to survive has developed over billions of years, since the time when our planet was a ball of swirling hot gases. As millions of years passed, the gases coalesced, forming a ball of hot liquid with a hard crust— the earth we know today. In less than a century—only an instant in relation to the age of our solar system—man has upset this balance through the creation of chemicals never before found on earth. He pours them into the environment with reckless abandon. The effects are already evident, and the point of no return may already have passed.

More people are alive today than the *total* of persons who have existed since man first appeared. In order to support this massive population, we have created machines and new chemicals. Most of these chemicals are beneficial, but a few are devastatingly harmful. The most dangerous are the ones that are still not recognized as harmful and the ones that, although known to be harmful, are still released into the environment because of the convenience of the monsters we ourselves have created: production, industry, and political expediency. These monsters may be our undoing, for unless they are controlled, catastrophic new plagues may eventually occur, caused not by bacteria, but by chemicals. Exposure of huge populations to potent cancer-causing substances, called carcinogens, and to other poisonous chemicals will likely be the death of us.

Our current standard of living is based on industrial production, and a necessary offshoot of industry is pollution. Factories foul the air and the streams, but they also provide jobs that give men and women dignity and the opportunity to live as good a life as possible. Antipollution devices can prevent or reduce pollution, but the devices are nonproductive and inflationary, as they add to the cost of the product. Politicians, who formulate the laws concerning pollution, must balance the needs of protecting the environment against the needs of industry to produce and to provide employment. Politicians also may have personal biases in favor of industry leaders who furnish campaign funds. The situation is a highly complex one that unfortunately has not been resolved in a way that assures protection from the dangers present in the environment.

During the evolution of our planet, when the landscape was being carved by glaciers, one area was uniquely formed. Two land masses emerged, perpendicular to one another and each surrounded on three sides by large, fresh-water lakes. Beautiful, large trees covered the land, and the air was pure. Glistening white sands lined the hundreds of miles of shoreline of the peninsulas. This was Michigan before it was inhabited by man.

It is now almost certain that man first emerged in Africa near the equator. Because he was able to adapt to and survive in varying environments and because he was forced to be mobile to maintain his food supply through hunting and gathering, man spread far beyond Africa. About seven hundred thousand years ago he reached Java, and four or five hundred thousand years ago he reached China and Europe. In China he was found as

Peking man, living in caves. These incredible migrations made man a widely dispersed species, even though his numbers were relatively few, perhaps one million.

Man migrated to North America from Asia not later than ten thousand years ago, and not earlier than thirty thousand years ago—toward the end of the last ice age. By this time the Great Lakes were formed, as were the physical boundaries of what is now Michigan.

The first people to inhabit Michigan were Indians. They respected the land, taking only what they needed to survive. They lived in harmony with nature.

Later the white man came. He cut down the trees, overpopulated the land, raped and despoiled the landscape, and built giant factories that belched smoke and chemicals—fouling the air and upsetting the delicate balance of nature. Animals began to disappear, unable to survive in the new environment.

Simon Pokagon, a Potawatomi chief and son of the man who sold the site of Chicago to the United States in 1833, told of his life as it once was:

> In early life I was deeply hurt as I witnessed the grand old forests of Michigan, under whose shades my forefathers lived and died, falling before the cyclone of civilization as before a prairie fire. In those days I traveled thousands of miles along our winding trails, through the unbroken solitudes of the wild forest, listening to the songs of the woodland birds, as they poured forth their melodies from the thick foliage above and about me.
>
> Very seldom now do I catch one familiar note from these early warblers of the woods. They have all passed away. . . .*

Michigan was a beautiful state. Parts of it are still beautiful, but the lower half of the lower peninsula is enveloped in a cloud of industrial and automotive pollutants. In addition to the usual industrial pollution and changes that occur with dense population, Michigan has fallen victim to several unusual and potentially catastrophic situations involving contaminants.

In order to illustrate Michigan's pollution problems better, and in order to show the kinds of problems that are occurring in

---

*From *I Have Spoken:* American History Through the Voice of Indians: compiled by Virginia Irvine Armstrong., Swallow Press, 1971.

many areas of the country, let's take an imaginary trip through the state. We will start in Detroit, the motor capital of the world. Detroit has a population of several million. It has one of the highest unemployment rates and one of the highest crime rates in the country. The amount of pollution from industry alone is exemplified by the fact that the Rouge River caught fire several years ago.

Let's now take westbound I-94 out of Detroit—past Ann Arbor and Jackson—to Battle Creek, about two-thirds of the way across the state.

Just west of Battle Creek we will pass a large, towering structure about ten stories high, visible to the left of the road. This is the feed-mixing plant of the Michigan Farm Bureau Services, where massive amounts of livestock food were contaminated with flame-retardant chemicals called polybrominated biphenyls, or PBBs, during the mixing process.

From mid–1973 through mid–1974 the approximately nine million residents of Michigan consumed low concentrations of PBBs by eating animals and animal products contaminated by the feed. This incident is discussed in detail in Chapter 10.

Now we will continue our journey on westbound I-94 past Kalamazoo to Benton Harbor, on the coast of Lake Michigan. Twenty years ago Benton Harbor was a vacation haven for Chicagoans. They flocked across the lake in droves to enjoy the beautiful, clear water and to lie on the fine-textured, white sandy beaches. They would stand on the bluff overlooking the lake just north of Benton Harbor, breathe the clean air, and relax. Some went to the numerous small resorts in the area. Others owned cottages. Fishermen went out in boats or out on the pier in Benton Harbor and caught their limit of perch or lake trout. It was indeed a beautiful place.

Then came the oil spills, starting in the 1950s, when globs of black crude oil stained the white sands. The opening of the St. Lawrence Seaway introduced the eel-like lamprey and the alewife. The lampreys killed the gamefish, and the inedible alewives replaced them by the millions. Pollution from the steel mills and other factories of Whiting, Gary, and Chicago killed what gamefish the lampreys left by contaminating the lower third of Lake Michigan with industrial waste chemicals.

Let's now leave Benton Harbor and travel north on I-96 past Grand Rapids and continue north to Traverse City. This is the last vacation area in the lower peninsula that *looks* unpolluted and is within reasonable driving distance of Detroit and Chicago. The beaches are still white and the water is still crystal clear. The area is famous for its cherries as well as being a superb vacation spot. However, the cherries are produced by the latest agricultural methods, including the use of massive amounts of insecticides, which drain off into the streams and rivers, contaminating the fish.

Unfortunately, if you catch any of the coho salmon or lake trout while you're in the area, you had better not eat them. They all have levels of polychlorinated byphenyls, another environmental contaminant, as high as thirty times the current upper tolerance limit. That limit may be made more stringent now that it is known that PCBs cause liver cancer in rats.

Let's now travel eastbound from Traverse City to I-75. On the way we will pass the town of Kalkaska, a burial site for over 23,000 cows that had to be killed because they were contaminated with polybrominated biphenyls that were added to their feed by mistake at the plant we passed earlier.

We could take I-75 north, cross the "Big Mac" bridge—a hundred-million-dollar structure connecting Michigan's upper and lower peninsulas—and go into the beautiful, relatively unspoiled, sparsely populated upper peninsula with its tall silver-white birch and pine trees. The air is sweet and pure. There is no industry to spoil the atmosphere. We could drive along the southern shore of Lake Superior, the largest freshwater lake in the world, and enjoy the incredible scenery.

Why don't we take this trip, you ask? Because you would stop along the way and want a drink of water. The water there is probably not safe to drink. It is loaded with cancer-causing asbestos. You will learn why, later in this book.

Instead, let's head south on I-75. We can stop at the village of Clare, Michigan, for a cup of coffee. Clare is the "jumping-off point" to the clean areas of Michigan. If you look to the south you can see the "crud line"—the brown cloud hanging over the southern third of the state.

It is about a three-hour drive back to Detroit, and thus ends our trip.

Man, like other animals, has the remarkable capacity to develop from a single-celled embryo to a complex organism. Although man's intellectual abilities exceed those of other animals, most people never develop their intellects. The brain must be trained through education and discipline to take full advantage of man's unique capabilities. Basic survival needs, including food, shelter, and reproduction, keep most people from the goal of developing their intellect. Early man had to spend most of his time fulfilling such needs.

In our contemporary civilization, the majority still have to spend most of their time providing the basic necessities of life. On the other hand, extensive specialization and division of labor have allowed some people to pursue education to its fullest extent. These relatively few people have led us to the brink of a supercivilization. We have sent men to the moon and brought them back. We have programmed space probes to explore the far reaches of our solar system. We have cracked the genetic code, and may be on the brink of understanding the processes of life and death.

But this development of mankind is gravely threatened by one glaring fact—there are too many of us. Leonardo da Vinci once said that most men contribute nothing to the development of civilization. They only exist, and in the process are a detriment to society. They eat, produce wastes, and when they die leave a decomposing corpse behind. The statement is still true today, but on a much larger and more serious scale. Most people today consume vast amounts of our limited energy resources while contributing very little to the progress of civilization. In the process of using these energy resources, whether by driving automobiles or using modern machines or their products, they are in turn polluting the environment to a degree that threatens man's existence.

In short, there are too many people, too many machines. We have two choices. We can cut down on the number of people, reduce pollution to a viable level, and progress to our supercivilization, or we can continue as we are and eventually destroy the human race. The choice is ours.

The basic problem up to now has been our own ignorance. Until recently, we introduced thousands of new chemicals into our environment each year without the foggiest notion that some of them were detrimental to our health. Now we know that they are. The problem is still one of ignorance, because we do not know at what dosage levels these chemicals are harmful. Is it safe to eat, drink, or breathe small doses once in a while? Or will even minute exposure cause cancer or some other disease? If we continue to be exposed to such agents without limitation, the problem will be one not only of ignorance, but of stupidity as well.

We obviously cannot live in a pollution-free environment. Even if we abandoned our modern civilization and did away with man-made chemicals, we still would be exposed to pollutants. We would be exposed to them just from cooking food, and even if we ate everything raw, we would occasionally eat naturally occurring carcinogens in plants. We cannot get away from them, but we can sensibly limit our exposure to harmful pollutants and minimize the risk.

The spectrum of concern regarding chemical pollutants in our environment ranges from total apathy and ignorance of the problem to near hysteria with calls to remove every trace of every pollutant. To approach the problem realistically, one must realize that even primitive man was exposed to pollutants, including carcinogens. Not nearly so many existed then as we have today, but they were indeed in his environment. Living in a technological society exposes us to many risks that primitive man did not have to face. These include such things as being one of the 50,000 people killed every year in the United States while riding in automobiles. One the other hand, we don't have to worry about being eaten by wild animals as our forebearers did. The risks are still present, but they have changed.

In order for so many of us to survive so long and to enjoy the material goods to which we are accustomed, we have to contend with the risk of polluting our environment. The answer is not to regress to the level of cavemen, but through research to identify the potent carcinogens and other chemicals harmful to both fauna and flora and prevent the widespread exposure of large populations of humans, other animals, and plants to these chemicals. Some groups will be required to have contact with certain dangerous chemicals if we are to maintain our present standard of living. These people should be informed of the risk, given the opportunity to decide whether they should continue their exposure, and be compensated adequately for accepting the risk. The objective must be to prevent large-scale disasters such as the development of cancer in large population groups exposed to potent carcinogens in consumer products or industrial pollution.

The words written and sung so eloquently by John Denver are especially fitting:

> *There's a heavy smog between me and my mountain*
> *It's enough to make a grown man sit and cry*
> *It's enough to make you wonder*
> *It's enough to make the world roll up and die.*
>
> **John Denver***

The prophetic last line will come true unless we take the appropriate measures to reverse the current trend of massively defiling our environment.

---

*Eclipse by John Denver. © Copyright 1974 Cherry Lane Music Co. Used by permission. All rights reserved.

2
Chemical
Carcinogenesis

"It is time for the scientists to speak out
and inform the public."
—**Joseph K. Wagoner, NIOSH**

CANCER—the very word strikes fear into the hearts of millions. It is mankind's most dreaded disease.

The cancer statistics are staggering. In 1969, 323,000 Americans died from the disease. In contrast, America lost 292,000 men in battle during the entire Second World War. Even the number of auto accident deaths per year is comparatively small, averaging 50,000 to 60,000 Americans per year. In 1972, 610,000 new cases of cancer were diagnosed, and one million people were under treatment for the disease.

The economic impact of cancer is staggering too. In 1971 it was estimated that the direct and indirect costs of cancer, including hospital and medical expenses and loss of earnings during illness and during the balance of normal life expectancy, totaled $15 billion. Medical bills alone averaged between $5,000 and $20,000 per patient.

11

Scientists now know many of the agents which cause cancer, but a universal cure remains unknown. The disease is caused by exposure to certain chemicals and viruses and to radiation. At the New York Academy of Sciences Conference on Occupational Carcinogenesis in March 1975, it was estimated that 80 percent of all human cancers were caused by environmental agents with heredity and other as yet unidentified influences accounting for the remaining 20 percent.

Certain chemicals, called *carcinogens,* cause cancer, and they are being poured into the environment constantly. Industry pollutes the environment with them through industrial wastes and mining processes. Air pollution comes from waste gases and smokestacks. The consumer also is exposed to carcinogens in consumer products. These are only some of the ways we are all exposed to cancer-causing chemicals.

The cancers diagnosed today may be the result of exposure to carcinogens twenty years ago. For reasons not now understood, there is usually a long incubation period—15, 20, 30 or more years—between onset of exposure to a cancer causing chemical, and the appearance of the malignancy. For example, vinyl chloride polymerization plants started operating in the late 1930s and early 1940s. The liver cancers began appearing in the 1960s and 1970s. Experts in chemical carcinogenesis predict that, due to the thousands of new, untested chemicals introduced into the environment in the past twenty years, the incidence of cancer will soar to epidemic proportions.

On purely economic grounds, it would appear to be a good investment for government to sponsor additional research to try to identify the carcinogens in the environment and then limit exposure to them. Yet this consideration has not been reflected in federal budget priorities. Most of the money is being spent on diagnosis and treatment of cancer. The prevention of cancer deserves at least equal consideration.

The American citizen must be aware of progress in cancer research for two reasons: (1) for his own protection so he can limit his exposure to carcinogens, and more important, limit the exposure of his children, and (2) so that he can apply appropriate pressure on his legislative representatives to see to it that more attention is paid to the *prevention* of cancer.

Chemical carcinogens do not produce cancer immediately after exposure. Rather, the carcinogen triggers a sequence of events or a chain reaction that eventually results in production of cancer cells. Studies of cancer of the liver and other organs have shown that the sequence begins with an *initiation* step, when the chemical attacks the genetic components (DNA) of the cell and alters the structure of the nucleic acid. This initiation step may be quite short, a matter of hours or days. It is followed by a prolonged period of development called the latent period, during which new types of cells are created because of the changes in the genetic components caused by the carcinogen. The growth of these new cells eventually results in development of malignant cells. To better understand the initiation and latent periods, we can compare these processes to pregnancy. It takes only a few minutes to start the pregnancy (initiation), but it takes nine months for the baby to be born (the latent period). For this reason, certain aboriginal tribes have had difficulty relating the two events. For the same reason, however, we in educated societies have had difficulty in understanding how exposure to cancer-causing agents now can affect us twenty or more years later. Now we understand this concept.

Just as our bodies have reparative mechanisms to protect us against injury and invasion from foreign substances, individual cells also have protective mechanisms to repair genetic or "initiation" damage. Within the nucleus of each cell are "repair enzymes" which, if given enough time, will repair damage to the DNA. For example, if a carcinogen enters the nucleus of a cell and reacts chemically with the nucleic acid, changing its structure, repair will take place if the cell does not divide in the near future. However, if the cell divides before repair is completed, the changes in the genetic mechanism will be transferred to the new cell and its "offspring," resulting in a new clone of altered cells. The transitory or reparable damage will have been converted to permanent damage by DNA replication. It is for this reason that tissues or organs in a state of rapid growth or repair from injury are more susceptible to carcinogens than tissues or organs whose cells are in a resting state. This is also why fetuses, infants, and young children are more susceptible to carcinogens than are adults.

With some carcinogens, only one exposure is needed for new types of cells to develop and eventually result in cancer. However, with most carcinogens, repeated exposure is necessary.

The potential for a carcinogen-induced catastrophe is very real and very awesome. For example, suppose that the new polyethylene plastic "collapsible" bags used to feed babies their formula in place of the old-fashioned glass bottles were made from plastics containing a carcinogen such as vinyl chloride instead of the noncarcinogenic polyethylene. And suppose that one million babies were fed by this new method, and a small amount of the vinyl chloride leached out of the bags into the formula. If 1 percent of all the babies who were fed with the plastic bottles developed liver cancer fifteen or so years later that would mean 10,000 babies would be doomed to die before they were twenty years old. This supposition is based on the material's being only weakly carcinogenic! If there were a moderate carcinogenic effect from the chemical and perhaps 20 percent of the babies fed with the plastic bottles developed liver cancer, then 200,000 babies would die before the age of twenty. The thought is staggering, but it might have happened if polyvinyl chloride had been initially chosen to manufacture the bags instead of polyethylene.

Baby bottles made of plastic are only one of thousands of products that have only recently come into widespread use and have never initially been tested for carcinogenicity. It will take only one mistake—only one product that is widely used and is strongly carcinogenic—to cause cancer in millions of people.

Let's look at another new product—the plastic thermos bottle. One taste of water stored in one of these containers makes a person nearly choke. Chemicals leach out of the plastic into the liquid stored inside. These chemicals are plasticizers or other additives and perhaps some of the parent plastic basic component as well. Even after numerous washings and storage periods the water still tastes and smells unpleasant. There are no reports in the medical literature regarding the toxicity of many of the usual components of these containers with regard to possible carcinogenicity, teratogenicity (causation of birth defects), or mutagenicity (causation of mutations). Next time you go on a picnic, keep that in mind!

Let us now examine another product which is used by millions of people nearly every day and is theoretically a high risk in terms of long term toxicity—the ubiquitous, disposable white styrofoam coffee cup. It is well established that foods in plastic containers, especially soft plastic containers, become contaminated with chemicals used to manufacture the containers. Styrofoam is polystyrene—a plastic made from the chemical styrene. As with other plastics, small amounts of styrene become trapped in the plastic during the manufacturing process. When liquids are placed next to the plastic, some of the styrene is released along with other chemicals including plasticizers, into the liquid. These chemicals account for the slightly different taste of coffee in a styrofoam cup from coffee in a ceramic mug. Thus, the user of a styrofoam cup exposes himself to small amounts of styrene and other chemicals almost every day. There are as yet no published studies showing how much styrene one ingests with each cup of coffee or other beverage consumed from these containers. Manufacturers have not been required to study the problem. Yet it is known that styrene is metabolized in the body to styrene oxide— a chemical which is known to cause mutations in bacteria. It is therefore likely that styrene oxide is a carcinogen as well. Here we have a situation where the product has not been available a long enough time for the latent period to pass. If styrene oxide is indeed carcinogenic and if we ingest enough styrene from the containers to produce cancer, we could, in the future, have a disaster of monumental proportions, with man being the unwitting guinea pig.

We have considered only a few common products whose long-range effects on our health are unknown. There are literally thousands more that have never been tested. Industry and government have put us, the consumers, in a rather undesirable position. In many cases we have become the unwitting subjects of tests—human guinea pigs in experiments that will last twenty to thirty years for carcinogens and several generations for mutagens.

As implied above, potential long-range hazards posed by

environmental pollutants and drugs include birth defects and mutations as well as cancer. The formation of birth defects caused by various chemicals has been recognized for several decades, but it was not until the thalidomide disaster of 1962 that the general public was made aware of the problem.

Embryotoxic Chemicals

Many people consider birth as the beginning of life, yet birth is really just one of the transitions in the life of a human being. Other transitions include: from neonate to childhood, childhood to adolescence, and adolescence to adulthood. Life really begins at conception—the creation of a single cell with the remarkable capacity to divide and multiply in a complex series of operations to form a human being. During this process the embryo duplicates the entire evolutionary process, changing from a single cell to two cells to a ball of cells. Then specialization begins, each group of cells differentiating more and more, changing both structure and function to become organs. It is an incredibly complex series of steps that must occur in a particular sequence. A monkey wrench thrown into the works can either kill or deform the fetus.

At each stage of life a person is subject to certain diseases. Arteriosclerosis is peculiar to middle and old age. Infectious mononucleosis is peculiar to adolescents and young adults. Chicken pox is peculiar to children. Birth defects are peculiar to the fetus. Certain viruses and chemicals can interfere with the developmental sequence of the fetus, and the end result can be death or deformity. A well-known example of a chemical that does this is the drug thalidomide. A virus that will do this is German measles. We know of other chemicals and viruses that cause birth defects, and there are undoubtedly many others in each category that have not yet been discovered.

Birth defects, or congenital anomalies, are generally defined as structural (anatomical) abnormalities that can be recognized at birth or shortly thereafter and cause disability or death. In a less restricted definition, birth defects also include microscopic, biochemical, and functional abnormalities originating during the prenatal period. Scientists study the effects of chemicals that might cause birth defects by administering them to pregnant animals (usually rats or mice) early in pregnancy, then sacrificing the mothers the day before birth and examining the reproductive organs and fetuses. They note the number of abnormal litters, the number of abnormal fetuses per litter, the types and incidence of each specific birth defect found, the number of dead fetuses, and the weights of the various organs and total weight of each fetus. They may also allow some of the test animals to deliver their babies to look for defects that may manifest themselves only after birth or later in life. Obviously, these tests are both expensive and time-consuming. Studies by scientists have resolved that at least some chemicals that cause birth defects may also cause cancer.

In testing for both birth defects and cancer production, chemicals are administered in greater amounts than might be expected in humans following accidental exposure or following chronic low-dose exposure. This is necessary to discover the potential dangers from chemicals that have only weak ability to cause birth defects or cancer. For example, suppose a new food additive were weakly carcinogenic and produced cancer in only one of every 10,000 people exposed to a certain dosage level. If the scientist exposed only 50 rats (assuming rats and people were equally susceptible), chances are that none of the rats would develop cancer and the additive would be judged safe, allowing millions of people to be exposed. If the chemical had the same cancer-producing potential in rats as in humans, 10,000 rats would have to be exposed before one rat would develop cancer. In fact, in order to obtain statistically acceptable data to declare the chemical unsafe, many more than 10,000 rats would have to be tested.

Many chemicals known to cause birth defects or cancer react differently in different animals, and humans may be more or less sensitive than test animals. For example, thalidomide can cause birth defects in humans with a dose as low as one-half of a milligram per kilogram of body weight. The minimum dose necessary in other animals is much higher. Humans are 60 times as sensitive as mice, 100 times as sensitive as rats, and 700 times as sensitive as hamsters. Thus it is necessary to test chemicals for birth-defect and cancer-producing properties at several dosage levels, including those higher than usual human exposure levels.

An anesthetic agent was found to produce tumors in mice as early as 1943. Two scientists noted with surprise that the lungs of twenty-six out of twenty-nine young mice involved in certain experiments had multiple lung tumors. The animals had received only small amounts of radiation and an anesthetic during the experiment. The anesthetic, urethane (ethyl carbamate) had been injected as a single dose into the abdomen. The scientists devised a new experiment, giving only the anesthetic to the animals, sacrificing them seven and one-half months later and looking for tumors. They also ran a control group of animals, housed and fed identically to the anesthetic-treated group, but with no anesthetic given. Eight of nine experimental mice had lung tumors, while none of the control mice had them. The scientists then studied the effect of lower doses of the anesthetic, insufficient to produce anesthesia. Four and one-half months after treatment, four of eight mice tested had tumors, demonstrating that anesthesia was not an essential part of the tumor-inducing process.

The scientists then studied the effect of the anesthetic in a strain of mice that normally had a high incidence of lung tumors and found that the tumors occurred several months earlier than expected if the mice received urethane.

In 1947 and 1948 other scientists tried injecting urethane into pregnant mice to see what would happen to the offspring. The offspring had an increased incidence of lung tumors, showing that the chemical, when administered to the mother, crossed the placenta into the fetus and caused changes that were not manifest until later in the life of the offspring. This experiment showed that the lung tissue in the mouse is susceptible to cancer production from the time the lungs are formed early in pregnancy. It was one of the first demonstrations of *transplacental carcinogenesis,* i.e., that cancer-producing agents can be taken into the mother, go across the placenta into the developing fetus, and there cause cancer.

It was not known whether this process occurred in humans until recently. A number of teen-age girls in the Boston area developed a usually rare tumor of the vagina. These girls were studied in detail and were found to have one thing in common. During the gestation period, their mothers all had received doses of a synthetic estrogenic compound called diethylstilbestrol

(DES). DES is known to produce cancer in animals. This chemical is the first known human transplacental carcinogen. Undoubtedly there are other similar chemicals, drugs, and hormones. As of 1972 there were at least thirty known transplacental carcinogens in animals, and the list continues to grow.

It has been noted that many of these chemicals produce cancer in the offspring only if administered in the last half of the gestation period. If administered only in the first half, they may either kill the fetus or produce a birth defect. A Russian scientist has shown that rat susceptibility can be divided thus: (1) From days one through ten, with peak effects on days three through five and day nine, chemicals tend to kill the fetus. (2) From days eight through eleven, chemicals produce birth defects; and (3) from day ten through delivery, the chemical may exert its carcinogenic effect, producing cancer later in the offspring's life. He also found that different dosage levels may produce different effects. Higher dosages in the last half of pregnancy may produce birth defects. These rules do not always hold true, as some chemicals, even if administered in the first half of pregnancy, may produce cancer. The three periods of pregnancy outlined indicate the times during which the three possible effects—embryolethality, teratogenicity, and carcinogenicity—are most likely to occur.

It has been found that fetal tissue may be much more sensitive to the effects of a carcinogen than adult tissue, in some cases requiring only 1 percent of the dose necessary to produce cancer in the adult.

It is now obvious that certain chemicals administered to the mother during pregnancy can reach the fetus and interact with its tissues to somehow produce cancer later in life. This has disturbing implications. But even more threatening is the evidence now mounting that the risk of developing cancer from exposure to certain chemicals may persist for at least two generations.

As early as 1952 it was reported that administration of methylcholanthrane (MCA), a known carcinogen, to rats both before and after mating resulted in tumors not only in the first generation of offspring but also in the untreated second generation. That is, the babies' babies also developed tumors. Other studies with other chemicals further confirmed this finding. This could be an explanation of why certain types of cancer run in families. It may also mean that the daughters of the girls who developed vaginal cancer may be high risks for developing the same disease. Other possibilities are that mothers who received DES may themselves risk developing the tumor, and their daughters will be high risks for the remainder of their lives. Furthermore, this rare type of vaginal cancer may not be the only type of tumor to develop, and other cancers may develop later in life.

According to international statistics, cancer in children has been increasing in recent years. In many countries it is the second most common cause of death in children, surpassed only by accidents. Leukemias and lymphomas (cancers of the lymph glands) are the most frequent types, followed by tumors of the nervous system and kidneys. These four types of cancer account for more than 80 percent of all tumors in children between eight and fifteen years of age. Scientists suspect that many childhood cancers were caused during the prenatal (or intrauterine) period by exposure of the mother to chemicals, drugs, or radiation.

The implications of transplacental carcinogenesis in man must not be underestimated. The studies in this area show the need to protect children and pregnant women from exposure to carcinogens. We are past the point where we can allow industry, lobbyists, and pressured bureaucrats to decide what our levels of exposure to carcinogens will be. It is time to listen to the scientists who know the truth regarding the tremendous consequences we face unless rather extreme measures are implemented soon. Otherwise we, and more tragically, our children and their children, will have to face the ultimate consequences of our stupidity.

Surprisingly, the theory that chemicals can cause cancer was advanced as long ago as 1775 by Sir Percivall Pott, an Irish surgeon living in England. He was sixty-two years old at the time and had practiced and taught surgery for twenty-nine years. He published a paper on cancer of the scrotum, which, he noted, occurred with some regularity among chimney sweeps. Historically, this was the beginning of cancer research. Pott made the point that the disease occurred almost exclusively among chimney sweeps and stated: "The disease in these people seems to derive its origin from a lodgement of soot in the rugae [folds] of the scrotum." By these words he described the first carcinogen known to man.

In his paper, Pott described the disease quite vividly:

> It is a disease which always makes its first attack on, and its first appearance in, the inferior part of the scrotum; where it produces a superficial, painful, ragged, ill-looking sore, with hard and rising edges.

He continued with the contemporary treatment of the disease:

> The trade [the chimney sweeps] call it the soot wart. I never saw it under the age of puberty, which is, I suppose, one reason, why it is generally taken, both by patient and surgeon, for venereal, and being treated with mercurials [a mercury-containing ointment used to treat VD in those days], is thereby soon and much exasperated.

He described the sociology of the disease as follows:

> The fate of these people seems singularly hard; in their early infancy, they are most frequently treated with great brutality, and almost starved with cold and hunger; they are thrust up narrow, and sometimes hot chimnies where they are bruised, burned and almost suffocated; and when they get to puberty, become particularly liable to a most noisome, painful and fatal disease.

Later on in his paper, Pott described surgery as the only hope of cure:

> If there be any chance of putting a stop to, or preventing this mischief, it must be by the immediate removal of the part affected; I mean that part of the scrotum where the sore is, for if it be suffered to remain, until the virus has reached the testicle, it is generally too late for even castration. I have many times made the experiment [surgically removed the cancer]; but though the sores after such operation have, in some instances, healed kindly, and the patients have gone from the hospital seemingly well, yet, in the space of a few months, it has generally happened, that they have returned either with the same disease in the other testicle or in the gland of the groin, or with such wan complexions, such pale, leaden countenances, such total loss of strength and such frequent and acute internal pains, as have sufficiently proved a diseased state of some of the viscera, and which have soon been followed by a painful death.

The disease Pott described is metastatic cancer of the scrotum.

Leading cancer researchers now estimate that as many as 80 percent of all cancers today are caused by chemicals in our environment. It is truly remarkable that Pott made this association two hundred years ago, before bacteria and the germ theory of disease were recognized.

Two major factors governing the production of cancer from chemicals are (1) genetic predisposition and (2) the latent period of carcinogenesis. Obviously, not everyone who is exposed to a chemical carcinogen gets cancer; otherwise the human race would have disappeared years ago. Some people are more susceptible than others. The reasons are still unknown but are ascribed to "genetic differences." The latent period of carcinogenesis refers to the usually lengthy time span between exposure to the chemical carcinogen and the production and manifestation of the cancer. In humans, the latent period can vary from several months to twenty years or more.

Even these basic concepts of chemical carcinogenesis were recognized early. Pott's grandson, Henry Earle, noting that not all chimney sweeps got cancer, wrote in 1823: "Constitutional predisposition is required which renders the individual susceptible to the action of the soot." He also mentioned that heredity and cancer are related, that scrotal cancer may appear in "different branches of the same family at a particular period of their lives."

Earle also noted that a latent period was involved in the development of the disease. He expressed difficulty in understanding why individuals exposed to soot as children did not develop the disease until after age thirty.

In 1808 a case was reported of one Allan Sprague, a forty-nine year old gardener who developed a skin cancer on his left hand. Five years earlier the man had had soot rubbed into the same spot on his hand, and the author suggested that soot may cause cancers in places other than the scrotum.

As early as 1892 another scientist, Henry Butlin, wrote in the *British Medical Journal:*

> We who live in large cities swallow and inhale soot every day in greater or less quantity. We accept the position, grumblingly no doubt, still we accept it: we know that our great smoke fogs make many people ill, and that they kill a certain number with acute

disease. But it is possible that we owe far more than this to the influence of "floating soot" and that a part of the increase in the occurrence of that awful disease, cancer, of which the national statistics tell so striking a tale, is due to the daily contact of soot with the lining of the mucous membrane, or to the entrance of soot into some one or other of the internal organs, in which the conditions are favorable to its action.

By this time other carcinogens were recognized, including tar, paraffin, and certain mineral oils. Butlin brought up another important question. Since these chemicals cause cancer of the skin, is it not feasible that they can also cause cancer of the internal organs?

Despite the early association between soot and skin cancer, it was not until much later that the first experimental confirmation of the relationship took place. Tumors were produced in rabbits at sites where coal tar had been painted on the skin. The work was performed by two Japanese scientists who published the work in the *Journal of Cancer Research* in 1918.

Tumor production by the first pure chemical carcinogen was demonstrated in 1930. Since that time many chemicals have been isolated and identified as carcinogens.

The importance of avoiding exposure to harmful chemicals is a lesson that has to be taught again and again. This very exposure has led to the discovery of new carcinogens in man, who has repeatedly been the unwitting guinea pig. Most human carcinogens have been identified from the occurrence of outbreaks of certain types of cancers in groups of workers in similar occupations or environments, followed by identification of the offending agent in the laboratory. The time has come for man to use mice and rats instead of human populations as the test subjects.

3
Occupational
Cancer

"Mother Nature has played a dirty trick on us."
—Irving J. Selikoff, M.D.

Occupational diseases have been described since antiquity. Hippocrates described lead colic as well as other toxic properties of this metal. Galen noted diseases peculiar to miners, tanners, fullers (cloth workers), chemists, and others. The Sallier Papyri describe the effects of certain occupations on ancient Egyptians. Pliny the Elder wrote that workmen in certain dusty trades tied bladders over their mouths to prevent the inhalation of dust. Other physicians and historians, including Agricola, Paracelsus, and Herodotus, discussed the influence of occupation on the health of the worker.

The first occupational cancer was described in 1775 by Sir Percivall Pott, as described in Chapter 2.

The first comprehensive textbook on occupational cancer was written by Dr. Wilhelm C. Hueper. The title of this pioneering work was *Occupational Tumors and Allied Diseases*. Hueper's contributions to the field were many. Born in Germany, he received his M.D. degree in 1920 from the University of Kiel and came to the United States in 1924. It was under Hueper's direction that the National Cancer Institute's environmental research program was inaugurated in 1948. Its activities included the planning of occupational cancer surveys, consultation services, and laboratory research. Much of the interest in the United States and abroad in the environmental causes of human cancer can be traced to the impact of Hueper's work. He retired from the National Cancer Institute in 1964. In 1975 he was honored as the first recipient of the newly instituted annual award of the Society for Occupational and Environmental Health.

Until recently the worker had little protection against development of cancer and other occupational diseases caused by exposure to noxious agents in his industrial environment. He was at the mercy of his employer's ignorance, carelessness or unconcern.

Passage of the Occupational Safety and Health Act of 1970 gave the worker the protection of the United States government. The Department of Health, Education and Welfare's National Institute for Occupational Safety and Health was formed and charged with identification of industrial health hazards. Since its inception, NIOSH has researched and published a number of criteria documents for industrial exposure situations and outlined the dangers involved and the adequate protective measures that must be employed. The Occupational Safety and Health Act of 1970 also provided for the formation of the Department of Labor's Occupational Safety and Health Administration. OSHA is charged with setting standards for safety in the workplace and with maintaining compliance with these standards.

The passage of the act and the creation of NIOSH was a great step forward in the history of occupational medicine. Among the industrial situations NIOSH has studied are occupational exposure to coke oven emissions, asbestos, arsenic, mercury, and a number of organic solvents. Current projects include investigation of vinyl chloride and anesthetic gases. Several of the exposure situations are examined in the following pages.

Coke Oven Emissions

Steel is the backbone of an industrialized society. The

tremendous temperatures required to produce it are created by burning "coke" in the steel furnaces. Coke is produced by heating bituminous coal to very high temperatures in huge ovens for up to twenty hours to drive off or evaporate the impurities. Coke is essentially pure carbon. Byproducts of this transformation of coal into coke include a wide variety of vapors and gases as well as tars and oils.

During the early years of steel production, until the start of World War I, coke was produced in "beehive" ovens that were used exclusively for the production of coke. The volatile matter produced during the process was emitted into the atmosphere. Newer ovens that permit the recovery of tars, oils, and chemicals from the volatilized portion of the coal were introduced around World War I, and by 1931 these newer ovens accounted for 80 percent of coke production. Today, about 95 percent of coke is produced with the recovery of by-products. Other methods of coal carbonization have gained recent popularity due to the energy crisis. Natural gas and other forms of energy can be recovered from coal by heating it to the proper temperatures.

The modern coke plant has three distinct work areas in terms of function and exposure of workers to the various chemicals: (1) the coal-handling area where coal is received and stored, (2) the coke ovens with equipment for charging and discharging the ovens, and (3) a by-product plant for recovery of gases and chemicals.

It is estimated that about 10,000 people in the United States work in the coke oven area of coke production. It has long been recognized that some of the products of both combustion and distillation of bituminous coal are carcinogenic. Early studies revealed that coal-tar products cause skin cancer, and more recent studies implicate coal-tar products and coke oven emissions in the production of cancer of other organ systems.

The history of the discovery of scrotal cancer among English chimney sweeps was discussed earlier. Since that discovery, the evidence has accumulated that workers engaged in the carbonization of bituminous coal and exposed to its products have increased risks for developing scrotal and other skin cancers. An early epidemiologic study showed the average annual scrotal cancer death rate among coke oven workers to be five times the rate for the general population. This study covered the period from 1911 to 1938.

The first report of a high incidence of lung cancer among these workers came from Japan. It was found that men working in the area where gas is produced in the coal carbonization process had a lung cancer mortality rate thirty-three times that observed among other Japanese steelworkers. This excess lung cancer risk was confirmed in a British study of the death certificates of steelworkers who died between 1921 and 1932. This study also revealed a high incidence of lung cancer among workers in other areas of coke production, especially among gas stokers and coke oven chargers.

More recent reports confirm the earlier studies. A 1952 study of retired gas retort workers demonstrated an incidence of lung cancer that was 81 percent greater than that observed in the general population. A study in 1971 revealed that coke oven workers in Allegheny County, Pennsylvania, had a lung cancer rate two and one-half times that of steelworkers in general. Another recent study of men employed at coke plants between 1951 and 1955 in both the United States and Canada confirmed these findings.

Other types of cancer have been reported as occurring more frequently among coke workers than in the general population. A high incidence of bladder cancer was reported among workers as early as 1931. The study reviewed bladder cancer deaths from 1921 to 1928 and reported a high incidence of this disease among occupational groups exposed to coal gas, tar, and pitch. More recent studies of British gas retort workers also showed an excess of bladder cancers among the workers, and it was suggested that the tumors were caused by exposure to the chemical beta-naphthalamine at the gas retorts. In another study coke oven workers in the United States were found to experience a higher than expected incidence of kidney cancers. Other studies also indicate high rates of cancer of the larynx, nasal sinuses, pancreas, stomach, and blood-forming organs (leukemia) among these workers.

Coke oven emissions themselves have not been tested for carcinogenicity in experimental animals. However, many of the individual chemicals produced in the manufacture of coke have undergone thorough testing. The cancer-producing properties of coal tar have been known since 1918, when Japanese scientists produced skin cancer in rabbits by painting the material on the animals. Benzo (a) pyrene is one chemical found in coal tar that has been identified as a carcinogen. In fact, this chemical is frequently used by scientists to produce tumors in animals. The potent bladder carcinogen beta-naphthalamine is also found in coal tar. Other chemicals that are known to produce skin cancer and that are found in coal tar include benz (a) anthracene, phenanthrene, and the "azo" compounds 4-amino 2,3-azotoluene, 2,3-azotoluene, and p-dimethylamino azobenzene. Coal tar also appears to contain a number of cocarcinogens.

Inhalation studies have shown that animals exposed to atomized coal tar developed lung cancer of the squamous cell type. This and other studies demonstrating the carcinogenicity of coal tar components in animals, along with the epidemiologic studies, leave little doubt that coal tar and some of its components are human carcinogens.

In 1973 the National Institute for Occupational Safety and Health published a criteria document recommending standards for occupational exposure to coke oven emissions. These standards include strict regulation of working conditions, including the use of special respirators and periodic health examinations for workers exposed to the emissions.

As a result of the NIOSH criteria document, the Labor Department has proposed new standards for controlling exposure of steelworkers to the cancer-causing emissions from coke ovens. It is estimated that the new standards could cost industry as much as $500 million in new capital investment and $295 million in additional annual costs.

Asbestos

Man has been using asbestos for centuries. The adverse biological effects of asbestos were observed as early as the first century by the Greek geographer Strabo and by the Roman naturalist Pliny the Elder, both of whom mentioned in passing a sickness of the lungs in slaves whose occupation was to weave asbestos into cloth.

Asbestos is a term that applies to a number of naturally occurring chemicals that contain the elements silicon and oxygen combined with water. A number of different metals also are present in the molecules of the various forms of asbestos. These chemicals will not burn, and they exist in the form of small strands, or filaments. There are various forms of asbestos. The type most widely used in industry is chrysotile asbestos, made of magnesium oxide and silicate, complexed with water.

Asbestos is widely used in the construction industry. It is also utilized in such products as textiles, brake linings, plastics, paints, and miscellaneous products. Almost one million tons of asbestos are used in the United States each year.

Most of the half-million tons of asbestos used yearly in the construction industry is incorporated into building materials such as floor tiles, shingles, and cement. The remainder is in "loose" form as insulation and acoustic materials, and the fibers can escape into the air and be inhaled. A few workers in the construction industry are particularly exposed due to the spraying of asbestos insulation materials, a technique that generates a great number of asbestos fibers in airborne particles.

Although there are only about 80,000 insulation workers exposed to asbestos dust in the United States, it is estimated that from three to five million other construction and shipyard workers are secondarily exposed to asbestos. Another 50,000 workers are exposed in the manufacture of asbestos-containing products.

Large-scale industrial exposure to asbestos did not begin until the end of the nineteenth century. The first case of asbestosis was recorded in England in 1906. The first complete description of the disease appeared in the *British Medical Journal* in 1927. The first case reported in the United States appeared in the medical journal *Minnesota Medicine* in 1930.

Asbestosis, which is noncancerous, is caused by the inhalation of asbestos fibers. Long-term inhalation causes a diffuse, chronic inflammation and scarring in the lung. The disease is manifested by (1) fibrosis, or thickening of the lung tissue, which can be seen on X-ray examination of the chest, (2) a crackling sound in the lungs, which can be heard during examination of the chest with a stethoscope, and (3) physiolgical changes consistent with a lung disorder. There is usually a considerable time lapse between initial inhalation of asbestos and the onset of changes in the lungs observable on X-rays. Examination of the sputum of patients with asbestosis reveals the presence of "asbestos bodies." These can also be seen in lung tissue taken during either biopsy or autopsy.

A study published in 1955 revealed a high incidence of lung cancer among British workers engaged in the manufacture of asbestos. Several years later similar findings were reported among workers in the United States engaged in the installation of asbestos insulation. Other studies revealed a higher-than-expected rate of malignancies of the gastrointestinal system and other parts of the body among asbestos workers. These findings came from studies of insulators, and pipe-coverers, and employees at an asbestos factory making both textile and insulation materials. The most highly suspect form of asbestos was the chrysotile, type, but amosite and other types were also suspect.

One particular type of cancer that occurs with some frequency among asbestos workers is called mesothelioma. It is a tumor of the lining of the lungs and peritoneum. Most cases of mesothelioma are in some way related to asbestos exposure. More than eighty percent of the cases studied in England and South Africa have been associated with asbestos exposure. In one study of 623 asbestos workers from 1943 to 1974, 444 men died, 35 of mesothelioma. Thus, almost one of every ten deaths was due to this tumor, which in the absence of asbestos, causes only one in ten thousand deaths. Other studies have confirmed the relationship between asbestos exposure and the development of mesothelioma.

It is now apparent that much *less* exposure to asbestos is needed to produce cancer than to produce asbestosis. A number of cases of mesothelioma have been reported among workers in the absence of X-ray changes typical of asbestosis. In fact, minimal exposure may cause mesothelioma. This has been illustrated by several reports of cases of mesothelioma among family contacts of asbestos workers, whose only contact with asbestos was with the dust brought home on the workers' clothes, and even among people living in the neighborhood of an asbestos factory, without any of the family members working at the plant.

In one "family" case a mother developed mesothelioma by washing the contaminated overalls of her three daughters who all worked for an asbestos company.

In another study of the development of mesothelioma among asbestos workers, the length of time between onset of exposure and development of the malignancy was examined in 344 worker deaths from all causes. Of the 344 deaths, 59 were due to lung cancer, 4 to mesothelioma, 18 to gastrointestinal cancer, and 31 to other cancers. Cancer deaths totaled 112. Twenty-four others died from asbestosis, while the remaining 208 died from other noncancerous causes. It appeared from this study that it takes longer (at least twenty years) to develop mesothelioma than it does to develop asbestosis (as little as ten years or less).

In another study, four cases of mesothelioma were reported among men and women with less than ten years of exposure to asbestos, and one of them had had only seven months of exposure. However, the latent period necessary for the development of the tumor ranged from twenty-three to fifty-three years. The latent period for development of mesothelioma in children is shorter, as cases have been seen in children under the age of nineteen.

It has been noted that mesotheliomas do occur among patients with asbestosis. But in most cases of mesothelioma, asbestosis is not seen. It has been postulated that long periods of exposure are required to produce asbestosis, while mesothelioma can be caused by short, intensive exposure, but it takes longer for the latter disease to develop.

At present it is still unclear whether one type of asbestos will produce more tumors than another. Studies show that all kinds of asbestos produce cancer. Some cause more lung cancer than mesothelioma and others tend to make mesothelioma more striking as a cause of death. For the affected person, either death is equally painful.

Further evidence that exposure to relatively small concentrations of asbestos can cause mesothelioma is seen in the case of a thirty-one-year-old man who developed the disease. His only exposure was from his father who, at age sixty-eight, had severe asbestosis from occupational exposure as a pipe lagger in Scotland. No precautions were taken to protect the family from contaminated work clothes, which were washed at home. Another case was reported in a man whose only exposure was from sanding floor tile containing asbestos prior to installation of a new floor covering.

It has been impossible to pinpoint a safe level of exposure to asbestos. From the case reports cited, it appears that even minimal exposure can be harmful to some workers.

Dr. Irving J. Selikoff has been the leader in research on the dangers of asbestos. He is the director of the Environmental Sciences Laboratory at Mount Sinai School of Medicine in New York.

"The reason it has taken so long to discover the link between asbestos and cancer," Selikoff explains, "is that Mother Nature has played a dirty trick on us." He continues by saying that until recently we have associated a disease with exposure to a chemical only if the disease is manifest within a few hours or days of exposure. With carcinogens, the latent period may be as long as twenty or even forty years or more. It is hard for people to accept this concept.

In a 1975 issue of the journal *Science,* Selikoff and his group reported the results of one of their recent studies. Analysis of fifteen samples of spackling, patching, and jointing compounds purchased in New York City revealed that five contained appreciable amounts of asbestos. The researchers concluded that the use of these materials in home repair work may expose the user and other members of the household to significant concentrations of asbestos.

In August 1975 the National Institute for Occupational Safety and Health expressed concern about exposure to asbestos among workers engaged in the maintenance and repair of automobile and truck brake linings. Researchers (the Mount Sinai scientists) had discovered that particularly large amounts of asbestos dust were created in maintenance shops where the large asbestos brake linings of trucks and buses were ground to fit the brake drum or were resurfaced after use. It was noted that the changing of asbestos brake linings for automobiles also was dangerous, because mechanics usually use an air hose to blow out the loose dust after removing an old lining. NIOSH estimated that as many as 900,000 workers are currently exposed to asbestos in the manufacture and servicing of brake linings and clutches. Most of these workers are auto mechanics. The agency recommended that repair shops designate a segregated area for all brake and clutch work and that signs be posted in those areas pointing out the dangers of asbestos dust. It recommended that repairmen wear respirators when doing such work and that strong vacuum cleaners be used to remove asbestos dust from brake drums before anyone works on them.

Although man has used asbestos for thousands of years, we have only very recently discovered the hazards of this material for both worker and consumer. Considerable research must be conducted before we will understand the full scope of the problems. For example, the effect of large amounts of asbestos in our drinking water is not yet known, but its presence remains a potential danger (see Chapter 12).

Bis (Chloromethyl) Ether

History is filled with episodes of man's inhumanity to man. One would hope that with civilization and technology would come recognition of human misery and efforts to alleviate it, but such does not appear to be the case. In fact, the advent of the industrial revolution brought about a new parameter of human abuse—abuse of the worker. Unfortunately, even in the space age, this abuse continues. An infamous episode that will live in industrial history is the story of Rohm and Haas.

The Rohm and Haas incident was well summarized in a report made to the Senate Subcommittee on the Environment, Senate Commerce Committee, by a determined young woman named Andrea Hricko, who represented the Ralph Nader-backed Health Research Group. She gave the report to the subcommittee on March 3, 1975, during hearings on the proposed Toxic Substances Control Act.

Ms. Hricko concentrated her report on the use of the chemical bis (chloromethyl) ether (BCME) at the Rohm and Haas chemical plant in Philadelphia, Pennsylvania. Since 1962, twenty-five workers exposed to BCME in just one building of the Rohm and Haas plant had died from lung cancer. This was at least eight times the expected rate. Although the corporate management suspected in 1965 and had sound evidence by 1967 that the chemical was a potent cancer-producing substance, the workers were told nothing about the dangers until 1971. Even then, they were told only that the chemical could cause cancer in animals. Regulatory agencies were not notified of the human cancer cases until 1974.

Ms. Hricko went on to summarize the chronology of events leading to the death of the twenty-five workers, pointing out instances in which adequate legislation would have altered the course of events and reduced the danger.

During the 1940s Rohm and Haas's Philadelphia, Pennsylvania, plant began handling the chemical chloromethyl methyl ether (CMME), which is always contaminated with BCME. Chloromethyl methyl ether is used in the manufacture of ion exchange resins. Full-scale commercial production began in the 1950s.

About twenty years after Rohm and Haas workers were first exposed to BCME, the company began to recognize that young workers in one building were dying from lung cancer. Three workers in their thirties became victims in one year. Because the company was suspicious of the chemicals used in the building, in 1962 it began a study of lung cancer among the plant's workers. Three years later Rohm and Haas contacted Dr. Norton Nelson of New York University Medical Center's Institute for Environmental Medicine to discuss the study of the carcinogenicity of a number of chemicals suspected to cause lung cancer, but Nelson was unable to reach agreement with the company on the contract. The dispute apparently was over the rights of the scientists to publish the results of the studies. Rohm and Haas demanded the right to withhold information from publication in scientific journals. Apparently because of this disagreement, New York University did not perform the study for Rohm and Haas. The company then contracted with Hazelton Laboratories in Falls Church, Virginia, to perform the studies. The contract fulfilled Rohm and Haas's demands on publication rights.

Dr. Benjamin Van Duuren, an organic chemist at the Institute for Environmental Medicine (the group originally approached), believed that, based on chemical structure, BCME and CMME might be the causative agents. On his own, he performed studies on these chemicals and confirmed his suspicions. The chemicals proved to be potent skin carcinogens in tests on rodents. Van Duuren and his coinvestigators recommended that "extreme caution be exercised in the use of these chemicals." This work was published in the *Archives of Environmental Health* in April 1968. The title of the article was "Alpha-halo ethers: A new type of alkylating carcinogen." Van Duuren's warning went unheeded at the time.

By 1967 the Hazelton studies had demonstrated an increased risk of lung cancer in animals exposed to the chemicals, and nine workers had died from lung cancer by this time. Workers and government agencies were not notified of any of the evidence, and even the medical scientists who had conducted the study were not given full information by the company on the work histories of the cancer victims. As a result, they did not realize the high incidence of lung cancer among the workers exposed to BCME. This alarming information remained the exclusive possession of Rohm and Haas executives.

Furthermore, new workers continued to be exposed to the chemicals. Finally, in 1969, the results of the Rohm and Haas–sponsored study showing that tumors developed in mice following injection of BCME were published. Rohm and Haas failed to make public the finding that inhalation of BCME had also caused lung tumors in mice. This was a crucial omission, because the workers were also exposed by inhalation. The publication also neglected to mention the fourteen cases of lung cancer that had been diagnosed among BCME workers by 1969.

In 1971 the plant was temporarily closed for modifications to reduce worker exposure to BCME. This followed an announcement by the Institute for Environmental Medicine that BCME was "the most potent cancer-causing substance ever tested" in the institute's nineteen years of lung cancer research. At that point—six years after Rohm and Haas first suspected and four years after the company had laboratory evidence that the chemical was carcinogenic—workers were told by the corporate management that the chemical was known to produce cancer in animals. However, even then the workers were not told that twenty employees in their own building had already developed lung cancer.

Also in 1971 the state of Pennsylvania adopted strict regulations for nine cancer-producing substances but did not include BCME. Rohm and Haas had not informed the state of the increased incidence of lung cancer among its employees.

By early 1972 an environmental newsletter carried the first published account implicating BCME as a cause of lung cancer in humans. The newsletter cited four cases of lung cancer in young workers who had been exposed to the chemical at a Diamond Shamrock plant in Redwood City, California. By 1972 twenty-four cases of lung cancer had been diagnosed at the Rohm and Haas facility, yet the scientific community was told nothing.

During 1972 and 1973 both the National Institute for Occupational Safety and Health and the Department of Labor's Occupational Safety and Health Administration (OSHA) published notices requesting information on the hazards of BCME and CMME, since OSHA was planning to set occupational health standards for these chemicals. Rohm and Haas responded to both notices. Each time, however, the company neglected to disclose to the government voluntarily that there was an increased incidence of lung cancer among exposed workers at their plant.

Ms. Hricko pointed out that during their investigation in 1974, Health Research Group representatives contacted many workers and families of workers from the Rohm and Haas plant. Many of them told of conditions in the plant during the 1960s, but they were reluctant or refused to give their names because they feared reprisals by the company. Many were bitter about what had happened to their fellow workers at the company and the way the company withheld data, but they were afraid to question the company about its policies. They feared being labeled "troublemakers" and possibly losing their jobs.

Ms. Hricko said that these Rohm and Haas workers need never have died from exposure to bis (chloromethyl) ether. If there had been mandatory provisions for premarket testing of chemicals with required reporting of adverse health effects, these twenty-five untimely deaths—and untold others in the future at Rohm and Haas and other companies—could have been prevented. It is clear that leaving the testing of toxic substances to the voluntary compliance and "good faith" of corporate management is more likely to result in experimentation on workers than in tests on laboratory animals. The chemical industry claims that these premarket testing provisions are too costly for the industry to bear.

The course is clear. Unless our government passes a strong toxic substances control act, every man, woman, and child in the United States will be at the mercy of irresponsible and unscrupulous corporate executives who can produce and market toxic products and/or expose workers to toxic substances. The case of Rohm and Haas could be just the tip of the iceberg.

Vinyl Chloride

In 1937 the B. F. Goodrich Company developed a process for making polyvinyl chloride (PVC) plastic from vinyl chloride gas. The Goodrich process is still in use today. It consists of piping vinyl chloride gas into large reactor vessels where the gas is agitated and mixed with a liquid and catalysts, causing the molecules of vinyl chloride to hook together and form chains. The product is the plastic we know as PVC.

After each batch of PVC is removed from the reactor vessels, a worker must crawl into the reactor and chip off the remaining PVC stuck to the sides of the vessel. The job requires about an hour, and a worker may be required to perform this task several times a day. While inside the vessel, the worker inhales considerable amounts of the sweet-smelling vinyl chloride gas.

The B. F. Goodrich plastics factory in Louisville, Kentucky, has been using this process since before World War II, making PVC for use as a fireproof coating for electric wire used in fighter planes and ships. Consumer products were being produced by the late 1940s, and during the 1950s PVC phonograph records and draperies were common household products.

Currently nine companies with fourteen plants and 940 employees produce vinyl chloride gas in the United States. The gas is made from a petrochemical, ethylene. The vinyl chloride gas is made into PVC by twenty-one different companies in thirty-six major plants employing 5,000 workers. About five billion pounds of PVC are produced annually in the United States, and about eighteen billion pounds are produced annually worldwide. There are between three and four thousand processing companies employing at least 350,000 workers who transform the PVC into hundreds of PVC products accounting for between $65 and $90 billion annually.

Toxic properties of vinyl chloride have been known since World War II. It was considered for use as an anesthetic but was rejected, fortunately, because of its myocardial irritant properties. In 1949 Russian scientists reported "hepatitis-like" changes in 25 percent of the workers at a PVC plant in that country. In the early 1960s toxicologists at the Dow Chemical Company reported that animals exposed to 100 parts per million (ppm) vinyl chloride developed liver damage. Because of these findings, Dow Chemical instituted a program to reduce factory air concentrations to below 50 ppm.

Another disease attributed to vinyl chloride was reported during the late 1960s. Skin lesions and changes in blood vessels leading to bone degeneration in the tips of the fingers and toes were found in some vinyl chloride workers exposed to high concentrations of the gas. This complex of symptoms in patients is called acroosteolysis. It is found mainly in workers who clean the reactor vessels and those exposed to high concentrations of vinyl chloride in the air. In 1970 University of Michigan scientists said that although they could not definitely prove that vinyl chloride was the cause of acroosteolysis, they recommended that the gas concentration be reduced to 50 ppm for industrial exposures. Except for Dow Chemical, which had already lowered its maximum permissible levels, the rest of the industry ignored the recommendations.

In 1970 Dr. Pier Luigi Viola, an Italian scientist, reported that levels of 30,000 ppm (3 percent) vinyl chloride was carcinogenic in rats, causing tumors of the ear canals, lungs, and bones. This was the first link between vinyl chloride and cancer. Dr. Viola later found tumors after exposure to 500 ppm. Further research on the cancer-producing properties of vinyl chloride was conducted by Dr. Cesare Maltoni, a researcher at the Institute of Oncology in Bologna, Italy. By October 1972 Maltoni had discovered that exposure to even 250 ppm vinyl chloride produced tumors of the ear canals and kidneys as well as angiosarcoma of the liver in rats.

Dr. John L. Creech, a Louisville physician who treated a large number of Goodrich employees, was the first to make the connection between vinyl chloride and angiosarcoma of the liver in humans. He had been concerned that a large number of Goodrich employees had liver disease. In addition to the nonmalignant liver problems, one of his patients, a Goodrich employee, had died of angiosarcoma of the liver in 1971. When another died in 1973, he suspected that something was terribly wrong, since the disease is extremely rare, striking only one of every 900,000 people. There are fewer than thirty cases per year reported in the entire United States. In December 1973 a third patient, a Goodrich employee for twenty-eight years, died of the same disease at the age of fifty-eight.

Following the three cases of angiosarcoma of the liver first reported by Creech, four additional cases were discovered among workers at the Louisville B. F. Goodrich plant. Three more cases were found at the Goodyear Tire and Rubber plant in Niagara Falls, New York, two cases at the Union Carbide plastics plant at South Charleston, West Virginia, and one case at the Firestone Tire and Rubber Company plant at Pottstown, Pennsylvania. Seven additional cases were reported from other countries.

Studies show that vinyl chloride workers have increased incidence not only of angiosarcoma of the liver, but of other cancers as well. A survey study of 8,384 vinyl chloride workers revealed that the workers, especially those with long exposure times, had an increased incidence of not only liver, but lung, lymphatic, brain, and urinary system cancers as well. A smaller study of workers at Goodyear's Niagara Falls plant found nine cases of cancer among 257 workers, while only four cases would be expected when comparing figures to the usual incidence of cancer in the general population.

It has been estimated that industrial sources may be releasing over 200 million pounds of vinyl chloride gas into the atmosphere annually from the vinyl chloride polymerization plants in the United States. Several cases of angiosarcoma of the liver have been found in people living near vinyl chloride plants, although the victims did not work in the factories. This suggests that very low levels from industrial emissions can cause the disease. If true, this fact would have tremendous implications for the general public.

We have all been exposed to small concentrations of vinyl chloride from aerosol spray cans and other consumer products. A spray can using vinyl chloride as a propellant, sprayed in a small bathroom for thirty seconds, can produce concentrations as high as 250 ppm.

Further studies by Maltoni have shown that concentrations as low as 50 ppm vinyl chloride can produce cancer in rats. In 1974 vinyl chloride was banned for use as a propellant in aerosol spray cans.

During May 1974 OSHA imposed a temporary emergency maximum permissible standard concentration for vinyl chloride, lowering the maximum permissible level from 500 ppm to 50 ppm. When it was later learned that even 50 ppm caused tumors in rats, OSHA, on October 1, 1974, lowered the permissible level to 1 ppm effective January 1, 1975. The new regulation actually states that exposure must be reduced to 1 ppm in factory air averaged over an eight-hour period, while up to 5 ppm may be tolerated over any period of up to fifteen minutes. Other groups are more conservative, stating that the only safe level is a zero detectable concentration. Controversy will undoubtably continue on this subject. Among the more conservative groups advocating lower or zero levels are NIOSH, the American Chemical Society, labor unions, and many medical scientists.

Although reports have been published concerning the carcinogenicity of vinyl chloride, until recently little information was available regarding the relationship between vinyl chloride exposure and the incidence of birth defects. Dr. Peter Infante, a dentist-turned-epidemiologist, studied the incidence of birth defects in several towns with polyvinyl chloride–producing plants and compared the findings with statistics from other towns.

Infante became interested in the problem after learning that Selikoff had noted in an earlier study that stillbirths and miscarriages among wives of vinyl chloride workers appeared to be two to four times the expected rate. Another report he had read demonstrated chromosome damage in vinyl chloride workers.

Because of these observations, Infante decided to perform an epidemiologic study of the distribution of birth defects in Ohio residents living in three communities that have PVC production plants. In addition to studying birth defects, he decided to include data on the incidence of cancer.

The three communities that have PVC production facilities are in the northeastern part of the state. Two cities, Painesville and Ashtabula, are located about five miles from the coast of Lake Erie. The third, Avon Lake, is about fifty miles west of Painesville. The populations of these three communities range from 12,000 in Avon Lake to 24,000 in Ashtabula. The PVC production plant in Ashtabula began production in 1954. The one in Avon Lake began in 1946. There are two plants in Painesville. One started production in 1946, the other in 1967.

For the four-year period 1970-1973, the number of children with birth defects and the rate per 1,000 live births were computed separately for each of the three cities as well as for the entire state of Ohio. For the entire state, the rate of malformations was 10.14 per 1,000 live births. The rates in the three cities with PVC production plants ranged from 17.37 in Ashtabula to 20.33 per 1,000 live births in Avon Lake. Painesville had 18.10 per 1,000 live births. The rates in all three communities were significantly higher than for the state in general. Infante then compared the rate in each of the three communities with the rates in the surrounding counties. Again, significant differences were noted.

The types of birth defects that occurred were of the central nervous system, upper alimentary tract, and genital organs. Club feet also occurred frequently.

The incidence of cancer, especially of the central nervous system, was higher than expected. The excess of central nervous system tumors occurred mainly in Painesville. Infante pointed out that Painesville also had a high rate of central nervous system birth defects among the offspring of its residents.

In his conclusions Infante stated that many factors could be responsible for the high rates of birth defects and central nervous system cancers in these communities, and the findings of his study obviously do not link polyvinyl chloride production with the maladies. But the findings do indicate a need for further study of possible contributing factors.

Trichloroethylene

Trichloroethylene, a chemical similar in structure to vinyl chloride, has widespread use. In the clothing industry it is used to dissolve plastic basting thread and to dry-clean finished clothing. A recent NIOSH study revealed that workers are exposed to high concentrations of the chemical when removing the clothes from cleaning machines. Other workers are exposed to high concentrations of trichloroethylene in electroplating processes, where the chemical is used to remove grease from metal surfaces prior to electroplating. Workers in industries using trichloroethylene are exposed to much higher concentrations of the chemical than the workers who manufacture it. Trichloroethylene is produced by five petrochemical companies. Production takes place in enclosed areas.

Like DDT, trichloroethylene is stored in body fat for long periods. When given as an anesthetic, it is measurable in the breath of patients up to twelve days following surgery. Although trichloroethylene is not a popular anesthetic at present, the number of anesthetics administered using this drug since its introduction is in the millions. One of its most popular uses until the mid-1960s was in obstetrical anesthesia using a device called the "Trilene Inhaler." The mother could administer the anesthetic herself whenever she needed it. The device fell into disrepute after several deaths occurred from overdose.

A study performed in Italy in 1971 showed that volunteers exposed to about 100 ppm trichloroethylene for four hours suffered impairment of their mental abilities, including reaction times and memory recall. A 1973 study revealed that concentrations of trichloroethylene up to 100 ppm occur in the operating room near the anesthesiologist while administering the chemical as an anesthetic. A rather disturbing thought!

The majority of the 600 million pounds of trichloroethylene produced in the United States each year is used in industry. However, some is used to extract substances from certain foods, such as in the production of decaffeinated coffee and the isolation of spice resins. It is also used in the processing of soy beans. The Food and Drug Administration allows a residue of trichloroethylene of up to 10 ppm in instant coffee and up to 25 ppm in ground coffee.

I met with Van Duuren in March 1974 to discuss the possible carcinogenicity of inhalation anesthetic agents. One of the most important areas of discussion was the possible carcinogenicity of trichloroethylene. We were concerned because of the structural similarity of this chemical to vinyl chloride, its route of metabolism, and its widespread use in industry and its less frequent use as an anesthetic. On our list of suspicious anesthetics, it was second only to the anesthetic isoflurane. (More about this appears in Chapter 14.)

In April 1975 Dr. Umberto Saffiotti, head of the carcinogenesis branch of the National Cancer Institute, revealed the preliminary results of the institute's carcinogenicity studies on trichloroethylene in an internal "Memorandum of Alert." Mice that were fed large doses of the chemical five times per week for eighteen months had a much higher incidence of liver cancer than control mice.

Although the studies were not conclusive and the finding was considered "preliminary," it is highly suggestive that trichloroethylene is carcinogenic, at least in high doses. The equivalent dose in man is about a shot-glass full per day. Further tests must now be performed to determine the effects of lower concentrations of the chemical.

Jane Brody, science writer for the *New York Times,* picked up the story and was the first to break the news to the general public. Saffiotti told her in an interview, "We learned a lesson from DDT, dieldrin, and other chemicals where the first data indicating a hazard was available years before action was finally taken to protect the public. The alert is a new type of action to keep us from sitting on a very important observation that may help people protect themselves from a cancer hazard."

He was referring to the several years that had passed between the discovery by Van Duuren that bis (chloromethyl) ether caused cancer in animals and the protection of workers from the chemical. It also took several years for workers to be protected from vinyl chloride.

Benzene

The chemical benzene has been used in various industries for a number of years. Benzene is used and inhaled by workers in rotogravure plants while using inks and solvents. In these plants benzene concentrations have been measured as high as 1,500 ppm. It is also used by shoe manufacturers as a solvent in glue. Concentrations of benzene where it can be inhaled by shoe factory workers has been measured and ranges from 25 to 600 ppm.

Benzene has been known for almost a century as a powerful bone-marrow depressant that leads to aplastic or hypoplastic anemia. Scientists now believe that chemicals capable of inducing severe bone marrow damage may also cause leukemia. Evidence has been accumulating over the past few decades that this association is true for benzene.

The first case of benzene-induced leukemia was reported in 1928. More than 150 cases of occupationally related benzene-induced leukemia are known at present. In many of these cases, leukemia developed as a terminal stage of a hyporegenerative anemia.

Aplastic anemia generally occurs in subjects while they are still exposed to high concentrations of benzene. Leukemia may occur at the same time or shortly after exposure. However, in a few cases, long latency periods have been reported. In a recent case a woman who had suffered from a typical anemia in 1957 after benzene exposure had had almost normal blood counts for the next fourteen years. She then developed leukemia and died five months later.

Benzene is also known to induce chromosomal aberrations, and this might be an important factor in the production of leukemia.

There are important implications for other workers and for the general consumer in the fact that the gasoline used in motor vehicles contains as much as 8 percent benzene.

Ethylene Dibromide

Ethylene dibromide (EDB), a chemical similar in structure to both vinyl chloride and trichloroethylene, has also been found to be carcinogenic to both rats and mice by the National Cancer Institute. EDB is used both in leaded gasoline as an additive and as a grain fumigant. An estimated 330 million pounds of EDB are produced annually in the United States.

Experiments conducted by the National Cancer Institute revealed EDB to be a potent carcinogen in rodents. The animals were fed various dosages of the chemical dissolved in corn oil. Seventy-six percent of rats tested and 87 percent of mice tested developed stomach cancer, some as early as ten weeks after the onset of the experiment. EDB is a highly irritating substance and has been known for many years to cause skin and eye injuries, respiratory tract inflammation, and even fatal heart problems. Accidental swallowing by humans has resulted in liver and kidney damage, but to date there has been no reported association between the chemical and human cancer.

The Ethyl Corporation is the largest producer of ethylene dibromide. Dow Chemical is another major producer. Both companies are currently reviewing the health records of workers exposed to EDB in their plants. Worker exposure is limited by law to 25 ppm.

NIOSH estimates that about 9,000 industrial workers are exposed to EDB during its manufacture or compounding with gasoline. An additional 650,000 persons employed in service stations are exposed to the EDB-containing leaded gasolines. Through its use as a grain fumigant, approximately 8,900 fumigators and exterminators also are exposed. Consumers are exposed on a massive scale to very low concentrations. Samples of commercially fumigated grains showed EDB residues ranging from 0.01 ppm to 6.10 ppm.

Although carcinogenicity of ethylene dibromide in humans has not yet been established, the National Cancer Institute study showing carcinogenicity in rodents dictates prudence in human exposure.

Chloroprene

The chemical chloroprene is a colorless liquid that is used to manufacture the synthetic rubber Neoprene. Neoprene is resistant to both weathering and oil. It is also resistant to abrasion, heat, flame, oxygen, ozone, and solvents. It is used to make cable sheaths, hoses, fabrics, adhesives, and a large number of rubber articles. The automobile industry is the largest consumer of Neoprene.

The duPont Company has used chloroprene in the production of Neoprene since 1931. In 1974 concern arose about the possible carcinogenicity of chloroprene because of its structural similarity to vinyl chloride. A search of the world medical literature revealed two recent Russian studies that suggested an increased incidence of skin and lung cancer among workers exposed to chloroprene in the Soviet Union. In addition, two other articles in the Russian literature described animal experiments in which the chemical adversely affected embryo development in both mice and rats.

Toxic effects from exposure to chloroprene have been known for some time. These include central nervous system depression and significant injury to the lungs, liver, and kidneys. Humans exposed to chloroprene have reported other symptoms, including dermatitis, corneal necrosis, anemia, loss of hair, nervousness, and irritability.

The Russian studies suggesting carcinogenicity of chloroprene involved a large-scale epidemiological investigation of workers in the Yerevan region. During the period 1956–1970, 137 cases of skin cancer were found among 24,989 persons over twenty-five years of age. This large group included both chloroprene-exposed workers and nonexposed workers. It was found that 3 percent of the workers with extended work exposure to the chemical had skin cancers, while only 0.12 percent of persons not exposed to the chemical had skin cancers. It was also noted that workers exposed to chloroprene-related chemicals had an increase in skin cancers.

The incidence of lung cancer also was studied in the same region of Russia. There were 87 cases of lung cancer reported among 19,979 workers in various occupations. Of the chloroprene-exposed workers 1.1 percent had developed the disease, while the rate for nonexposed workers was considerably lower.

It has been estimated that about 1,600 employees of E. I. duPont de Nemours & Company are involved in the production of Neoprene from chloroprene. Chloroprene is also made by the Petro-Tex Chemical Company in Houston, Texas.

Arsenic

Arsenic is a rather ubiquitous element. It is found in small amounts in soils and waters throughout the world as well as in a number of foods, particularly seafoods. It is also present in a number of minerals and is obtained for commercial use from the ores of metals, being present as an impurity. It is removed as the compound arsenic trioxide during the smelting of ores. In the United States arsenic is produced mainly from the smelting of copper ore. Arsenic trioxide is then used in the manufacture of most other arsenic-containing compounds for commercial use.

About 30,000 tons of arsenic trioxide are used in the United States annually. The various arsenic-containing compounds produced from arsenic trioxide include pesticides, pigments, and copper and lead alloys. Arsenic compounds are used in the manufacture of glass, textile printing, tanning, taxidermy, and lubricating oils. Numerous occupations have potential exposure to arsenic, and NIOSH estimates that 1,500,000 workers are potentially exposed to inorganic arsenic.

Chronic arsenic poisoning has been the topic of several classic murder mysteries. The initial symptoms are nausea, vomiting, diarrhea, hot flashes, and progressive anxiety. Similar episodes continue intermittently. With the passage of time there is a gradual darkening of the skin and a thickening of the skin over the palms and soles. Muscular weakness becomes apparent, and the extremities become numb. There is a gradual loss of vision. Transverse white lines occur in the nails. Finally, severe heart failure occurs.

Chronic arsenic poisoning has been reported in a number of

workers in several different occupations involving the use of arsenic compounds. At one time arsenic was considered a beneficial stimulant and was popular as a tonic. Another medication, Fowler's solution, contains arsenic and is used for treatment of psoriasis and other conditions. Chronic arsenic poisoning has been reported in patients using these medications.

In 1953 twenty-seven cases of cancers of the skin and internal organs due to arsenic were reported in the medical journal *Cancer*. Arsenic was considered to be the cause because all victims except one, exhibited signs of arsenic poisoning in addition to the cancers, and that one patient had been using Fowler's solution for treatment of psoriasis. In addition to skin cancer, malignancies were reported in the urogenital, oral, esophageal, and respiratory areas, and ten patients had multiple skin and internal cancers.

In a study announced in August 1974 Dow Chemical Company and Allied Chemical Company surveyed their retired employees and found those who had worked with arsenic during their employment had a frequency of lung cancer that was seven times the expected rate, and cancer of the lymphatic system occurred at six times the expected rate.

Allied Chemical supported its study through Johns Hopkins University. The study group found that of twenty-two deaths among retired personnel of a Baltimore plant using arsenic, seventeen were caused by cancer. Lung cancer accounted for ten of the deaths, while lymphatic cancer accounted for three more. The expected rate of death from cancer for the group was only 1.2 workers. This report, given by Allied Chemical to OSHA, followed a previous Allied study of twenty-seven deaths among employees and former employees from 1960 to 1973. Of those twenty-seven deaths, nineteen were due to cancer, again predominantly of the lung and lymph glands.

The Dow Chemical report also revealed high death rates from lung cancer and lymphosarcoma among employees who had worked at an arsenic processing plant that was no longer in operation.

As early as January 1974 NIOSH urged the Labor Department to reduce the maximum tolerable limit of exposure to arsenic in industry. It was recommended that air contamination be reduced from 0.5 milligrams per cubic meter of air to 0.05 milligrams.

When its study was released, Allied Chemical announced that all employees and retirees would be notified of the risks and that the company would assume medical costs for those afflicted. Company officials stressed the need for frequent medical examinations of those at risk.

Following their own sponsored reports, both companies have taken steps, without waiting for government regulations, to reduce employee exposure to as low a level as possible. Both Allied Chemical and Dow Chemical deserve credit for these actions.

Wood and Wood Products

Recent studies have suggested that occupations associated with the handling of wood in various forms have an increased risk of developing certain cancers. One such survey was conducted in the state of Washington by Dr. Samuel Milham of the Washington State Department of Social and Health Services. He reported his findings at the 1975 New York Academy of Sciences Conference on Occupational Carcinogenesis.

Milham studied the incidence of different types of cancer among various wood workers, including loggers, pulp and paper mill workers, plywood mill workers, sawmill and other wood machining workers, and carpenters.

The loggers, who work primarily in the forests, had an overall cancer rate that was low compared to that of the general population, but cancers of the stomach and prostate gland were higher than expected. Leukemias, especially lymphatic leukemias, also were somewhat higher than expected.

Pulp and paper mill workers experienced higher than expected rates of cancer of the small intestine and cancers of the lymphatic and blood-forming tissues. Lymphosarcoma, Hodgkin's disease, multiple myeloma, and lymphatic and monocytic leukemias all occurred at higher than expected rates.

Plywood mill workers showed increases in cancer of the stomach and cancers of the lymphatic and blood-forming tissues. In the latter categories, multiple myeloma, myeloid and acute leukemia, but not lymphatic leukemia, were reported at increased rates.

Only testicular tumors and cancer of the pancreas were noted in excessive rates among workers in sawmills and other wood machining operations.

Carpenters had an excess death rate from stomach cancer and Hodgkin's disease. Rates of multiple myeloma and leukemia also were somewhat higher than expected.

The fact that stomach cancer was increased in three of the wood-exposed groups suggests that ingested (inhaled or swallowed) wood particles may cause stomach cancer. The fact that cancers of the blood-forming organs were noted especially in the pulp, paper, and plywood workers suggests that the chemical and physical breakdown products of wood may be carcinogenic.

A major negative finding in Milham's study was that men who work in sawmills where wood is simply machined did not show the striking increase in malignancies that were seen in the paper, pulp, and plywood workers. He pointed out that the data suggest that these work environments contain carcinogens, but whether the carcinogenic agents are the woods themselves, chemical and/or physical breakdown products of woods, or chemical agents associated with wood processing or treatments remains to be studied.

It is interesting to note that in another study, furniture workers in England were found to have a high incidence of cancer of the nose and paranasal sinuses. None of the groups of workers in Milham's study had an excess of such cancers. In addition to geographical location, one major difference between the workers in the two studies is the type of woods to which the workers are exposed. The British furniture workers are exposed primarily to hardwoods, whereas the workers from the state of Washington are exposed primarily to softwoods. Furthermore, furniture workers may be exposed to a variety of paints and solvents that may contain carcinogens.

Formaldehyde

The largest industrial use of formaldehyde is in the manufacture of resins for plastic and synthetic fabric manufacturing processes. Some of these resins are used for thermosetting powdered plastic materials while others are used to treat textiles for their permanent crease and permanent press qualities.

Formaldehyde is also a powerful antiseptic, germicide, fungicide, and preservative that is used widely in the tanning and preservation of hides and furs, in embalming, and in the formulation of disinfectant, germicidal and fungicidal fluids. It is used to improve the fastness of dyes on fabrics, in waterproofing and strengthening fabrics, in processing and preserving rubber latex, and in preserving foods. It is also used in hardening paper and paper products, in developing photographic film, and in refining gold and silver.

Formaldehyde affects workers by causing irritation of the eyes, nose, mouth and throat. It has a very pungent odor that is offensive even in low concentrations, causing burning and tearing of the eyes. Higher concentrations cause difficulty breathing, intense burning of the eyes, nose and throat, and severe coughing. Prolonged exposure to high concentrations cause headache, abnormal heartbeat, and inflammation of the bronchial tubes and lungs. Wheezing may occur even at very low concentrations in some individuals. Dermatitis may occur from contact with skin.

Probably the most serious threat from formaldehyde in terms of long term risk is cancer. Formaldehyde reacts with hydrochloric acid in humid air to form the very powerful cancer-producing chemical bis (chloromethyl) ether, or BCME, which was discussed earlier in this chapter.

Kepone

Kepone, a white powder which is a potent insecticide against ants, roaches and potato bugs, was developed in 1951 by the Allied Chemical Company. The chemical was manufactured at various times in Allied's plant in Hopewell, Virginia, and by arrangement with other chemical companies in Niagara Falls, New York and State College, Pennsylvania. In 1974, Allied contracted with Life Science Products Company in Hopewell to produce the chemical. Life Science was a new firm started by two former Allied Chemical employees.

During the 1960s, investigations of the subchronic toxicity of Kepone in mice were reported. These studies showed that Kepone produced liver changes and damage to the nervous system manifested by tremors and ataxia. Deleterious effects on reproduction were noted at doses as low as five parts per million. These studies also alluded to the cumulative nature of the toxic effects of the chemical.

As early as 1961, Allied Chemical Company officials informed the FDA about Kepone's acute toxicity and later warned Life Science that the pesticide, which can be absorbed through the skin, should be handled with care. The warning went largely unheeded. Workers, unaware of the danger, neglected to wear the rubber gloves which were issued. Some ate lunches off tables covered with the chemical while others returned home covered with Kepone dust.

Workers developed slurred speech, memory loss, trembling hands, and pains in the chest and stomach. Tests revealed brain, liver, and spleen damage and some became infertile.

Kepone was tested in the National Cancer Institute's bioassay program. The studies commenced in November, 1971 and May, 1972 for mice and rats respectively. Both groups were fed Kepone in their diet for eighty weeks. According to the National Cancer Institute, the mice were killed after ninety weeks (August, 1973), and the rats were killed after one hundred and twelve weeks (July, 1974). The final results of the Kepone cancer study were not released until August 8, 1976—almost two years after the last experimental animals were killed. Scientists have been critical of this long delay, suspecting that if the results had been available earlier, Life Sciences employees' exposure to the chemical might have been shortened, thus reducing the risk of developing cancer or the other above mentioned disease conditions. Unfortunately, Kepone was found to be carcinogenic in rodents at doses as low as ten parts per million.

The Life Science plant was closed in July, 1975, because of the lax and sloppy conditions which allowed the workers to be exposed to the chemical. Since that time, doctors have treated more than seventy Life Science employees and their families for Kepone poisoning.

The problem may not be limited to the employees and their

families. For 16 months prior to its closure, the Life Science plant discharged its toxic wastes through the Hopewell sewage treatment system into the James River. Traces of Kepone have been found in fish and shellfish from the area and authorities have closed the James River and its tributaries from Richmond to the Chesapeake Bay to fishermen. In July, 1976, the Virginia Institute of Marine Science announced that Kepone had been found in bluefish taken from the lower Chesapeake Bay and warned that the insecticide could affect all parts of the bay.

The Kepone disaster occurred because of inadequate safeguards for protection of both workers and the environment. Similar disasters will continue to occur until preventive measures are enacted by our legislators.

It is encouraging that in October 1976, U.S. District Judge Robert R. Merhige fined the Allied Chemical Corporation and the Life Science Products Company more than seventeen million dollars. In addition, the two former Allied Chemical employees who founded Life Science Products, William P. Moore and Virgil Hundtofte, were fined twenty-five thousand dollars each and placed on five years probation. Before fining Allied Chemical, Judge Merhige called pollution, "A crime against every citizen," and he said, "the word must go out, we are not going to pollute the waters."

4
Chemicals in Your Food

"Eat, drink, and be merry, because tomorrow we die"
— G. J. Whyte-Melville

The next time you sit down to a Lucullan repast, consider what may be in the various epicurean delicacies you are about to savor. The pâté de foie gras may contain pesticide or antibiotic residues. The caviar may be loaded with polychlorinated biphenyls. For those with more plebeian tastes, consider the ignoble hot dog. It may contain not only diethylstilbestrol, but probably some sodium nitrite as well.

Nitrosamines

Scientists are concerned about the unnecessary use of large amounts of sodium nitrite in processed meat products, because the chemical can combine with other chemicals to form extremely potent carcinogens called nitrosamines.

There are three ways that nitrosamines can find their way

into our diets. First, they can occur in nature. Nitrosamines have been isolated from edible mushrooms, but these nitrosamines may not be the cancer-causing kind. Second, they may be formed in foods that have nitrate or nitrite preservatives added. Amine substances present in most foods to which the preservatives are added combine with nitrite to form nitrosamines. Hot dogs, sausages, lunch meats, most hams, and cured meats fall into this category. Nitrites also combine with the meat to form a red substance that makes the meat look fresher than it actually is. Hence meat packers, more interested in making a profit than in your health, add considerably more nitrite to the meat than is necessary for preservation, hoping you will buy it more readily because it looks better. Third, under certain conditions nitrosamines can be formed in our stomachs in the presence of gastric juice. The only requirements are that the nitrites and the amine substances be present. The amines are in most of the foods we eat; all we need to add are the nitrites. The necessary chemical reaction has been demonstrated in the test tube, mixing human gastric juice with the necessary components. The more acid in the gastric juice, the more readily the cancer-producing agents are formed.

The cancer-producing ability of the nitrosamines in animals is remarkable for its potency and versatility. In some cases only a single dose is necessary to produce a tumor. No matter how it is given—by mouth, injection, or inhalation—a dose of nitrosamine can produce tumors in a variety of organs. Obviously, humans cannot be used for laboratory testing of these agents, but there is no reason to suspect that we react differently from the rest of the animal world to the effect of these chemicals. Tumors are produced in all animals tested, including mice, rats, pigs, hamsters, fish, ducks, and others.

It is the responsibility of the Food and Drug Administration to curb the use of nitrite preservatives. The FDA appears to be lacking in its responsibilities. At an FDA hearing in March 1971, when nitrite additives were discussed, FDA officials testified that there is no need to lower levels of nitrite additives until more research is performed. On the other hand, a highly respected scientist, Dr. William Lijinsky of the Eppley Institute of the Nebraska Medical Center, disagreed sharply with FDA Commissioner Charles Edwards. Lijinsky, who has conducted extensive studies on the biochemical transformation of nitrosamines, stated that levels of nitrites should be reduced and suggested that they may not be needed at all in refrigerated meats, as their only function there is to sustain color. He did not discourage the use of nitrite in canned foods because of the danger of bacterial contamination without them. Lijinsky made the point that because of the potential hazard of the formation of nitrosamines in the stomach from amines and nitrites, addition of either or both should be severely limited.

At these hearings Lijinsky also expressed concern regarding the hazards of new drugs. Several hundred drugs now in common use are composed of secondary or tertiary amines. Under certain conditions these could form nitrosamines in the stomach, and some of the nitrosamines could be carcinogenic. Many of these drugs are of the type that are taken for long periods of time, including tranquilizers, antihistamines, and diet pills.

Unless the FDA curbs the use of these potential cancer-producing agents, it is remiss in its duty to the public. The FDA has the awesome responsibility of gambling with the lives of all the people in the country. If even the slightest chance exists that these chemicals are harmful, they should be curbed until proof is obtained that they are not harmful. The FDA appears to want to do it the other way—gamble that they are not harmful until proof exists that they are.

Research on the toxic effects of nitrosamines was begun after there were indications of liver disease among factory workers who were exposed in industry to the compounds. It was not until much later that it was suspected that nitrosamines occurred in areas outside the industrial environment. The first good indication arose when an outbreak of liver disease occurred in sheep in Norway. All the affected sheep had been fed a fish meal preserved with nitrite. Analysis of the meal showed the presence of dimethylnitrosamine, with concentrations as high as 100 parts per million in some samples. Pure dimethylnitrosamine given to sheep as a test produced the liver disease. This demonstration of nitrosamines in fish meal preserved with nitrite raised the possibility that nitrosamines might occur in foods preserved for human consumption. These concentrations may not be high enough to produce the acute toxic effect (the liver disease) but could be high enough to produce cancer if the foods were consumed for a long enough period.

Let's now look in more detail at the widespread occurrence of nitrosamines and their possible effects on our health. Numerous reports have been prepared regarding nitrosamines in food and drink, including smoked herring, kippers, smoked haddock, smoked sausage, bacon, smoked ham, and certain mushrooms.

In a Canadian study fifty-nine samples of various meat products were purchased at local stores and measured for levels of dimethylnitrosamine. Five samples had positive tests, including two different samples of salami and three different samples of dry sausage. In the samples 0.01 to 0.08 ppm were detected. Other scientists have shown that 2 ppm in the drinking water of rats for a period of 120 weeks produced liver tumors. A no-effect level in rats has not been demonstrated.

Samples of hot dogs from eight large manufacturers were analyzed for dimethylnitrosamine. Trace levels were found in the products of five of the manufacturers. Two of twenty-two samples from another producer were more highly contaminated. One sample of twelve from another manufacturer contained still higher levels. The highest level found in this study was 84 micrograms per kilogram of meat.

A high incidence of liver and esophageal cancer in parts of East Africa have been linked to nitrosamine-containing food and drink native to the area. In addition, the juice of a local fruit used to curdle milk has been found to contain nitrosamines. Another plant, used for medicinal purposes by the natives, was found to contain dimethylnitrosamine. The plant was used as a tea consumed for relief of stomach aches, and the crushed fruit of the plant was given in milk for the treatment of worms.

It is now a well-established fact that nitrosamines can form from nitrites and secondary amines in the presence of human gastric juice and acidic conditions with a pH of between 1 and 3. Feeding nitrites and secondary amines to rats has produced cancers.

Other studies have shown that certain agricultural chemicals—herbicides and pesticides—also can combine with nitrites under certain conditions prevailing in the human stomach to form carcinogenic compounds. Since nitrites are present in so many foods, a cancer hazard may exist in the residues of these pesticides and herbicides in our food.

The problem of nitrites in our food supply can be summarized by saying that in view of the natural occurrence of nitrosamines in foodstuffs and of their synthesis in the human stomach, there is a strong possibility that these potent carcinogens may be responsible for some forms of "spontaneous" cancer in man. There is an urgent need to determine the health hazard to man from trace quantities of these and other carcinogens in our food supply.

Diethylstilbestrol

Possibly the greatest risk from eating foods processed for mass human consumption is that of developing cancer from certain of the additives. Of special concern is the exposure of children to carcinogens because they are often more susceptible than adults and they have longer to survive the latent period. If a person fifty years old ingests a cancer-producing chemical and the lag period is twenty-five years, he may develop cancer at age seventy-five—near or beyond the end of his expected life span. However, if an infant or child ingests the chemical, he may be only in his mid-twenties when he gets cancer—a real tragedy.

One of the most disturbing aspects of modern beef production is the use of the chemical diethylstilbestrol, commonly abbreviated DES. It mimics the estrogen class of hormones and is used because it speeds growth and fattening of cattle. It is also used in the poultry industry. Studies indicate that if DES is withdrawn from the feed one week before slaughter, no residues will be present in the meat. However, many livestock producers give the hormone by injection in oil, which causes a slow release of the DES over a period of time, and the occurrence of residues in the meat is less predictable. Poultry appears to contain residues longer than beef or lamb.

DES is of concern because, as mentioned in Chapter 2, it is a transplacental carcinogen in man. This was discovered in 1971 when DES was found to be responsible for the development of aden'ocarcinoma of the vagina in a number of teen-age and young adult women. Their mothers had all received injections of DES during pregnancy as a measure to prevent threatened abortion. The latent period appears to be between seven and twenty-five years, although any woman whose mother received the drug must be considered at risk throughout her life.

We do not know what risk we run by eating low concentrations of DES in meat over a long period of time. But if one injection during pregnancy will cause cancer in the child, common sense dictates that it would be stupid to take the chance of eating small amounts continually. We may be lucky and find out that low concentrations are not harmful, but at the other extreme, we may find that a large percentage of people eating low concentrations for long periods of time develop an incurable form of cancer, such as cancer of the liver. We do not know the answer, and we are playing Russian roulette every time we buy meat in the grocery store. Much of our meat probably does not contain DES, but some does, and the sampling system is grossly inadequate to pick up the majority of contaminated meat. Officials of Canada, Australia, and other governments are concerned enough about the problem to ban the use of DES entirely from their own livestock production, and they have banned the importation of beef raised in the United States because DES is used here. With this information, we leave the subject of DES and hope you enjoy your next steak!

Red No. 2

The chemical amaranth, otherwise known as Red No. 2, is used as a coloring agent in solid foods, beverages, and pharmaceuticals in over sixty countries. Yearly consumption of this chemical for these purposes is over 1,500,000 pounds. In 1966 the World Health Organization Expert Committee on Food Additives determined that the dye could safely be consumed in quantities up to 1.5 milligrams per kilogram of body weight per day, or about 90 milligrams per day for an average-sized man. However, studies by Russian scientists in 1970 suggested that Red No. 2 had an embryotoxic effect in rats. An FDA study in

1972 showed a dose-related effect in rats on the number of live fetuses born per litter, indicating a specific fetal toxic effect. A greatly increased number of late fetal deaths also occurred. A study of the metabolic products of Red No. 2 showed that these substances also were toxic. In another study Red No. 2 was fed to rats in doses up to 30 milligrams per day for periods up to eighteen months. Growth was markedly depressed and mortality increased. Liver damage was demonstrated. The changes in the liver were similar to those seen in animals fed "butter yellow," a chemical that is known to cause liver cancer. The authors of this study suggested that the permitted level of Red No. 2 in food be reassessed.

In early 1976, it was announced that a study at the FDA's National Center for Toxicological Research in Arkansas suggested that Red No. 2 causes cancer when fed in high doses to test animals. This study appeared to support a 1971 Russian study which linked the dye to cancer production in test animals. The FDA study was challenged by the dye manufacturers association.

In late January, 1976, the FDA banned the use of Red No. 2, and manufacturers shifted to Red No. 40, another coal-tar based chemical which is approved by the FDA. Red No. 40 is similar in structure to Red No. 2, but it has not been adequately tested for carcinogenicity, and since it is not *known* to be carcinogenic, it has FDA approval. This is an inconsistent practice on the part of the FDA, since Red No. 2 was actually prohibited on the grounds that its safety had not been proved, rather than because it definitely was proven to be a carcinogen.

An interesting sidelight of the Red No. 2 story was reported in the medical journal *Pediatrics*. A young boy was admitted to a hospital after passing stools "looking like strawberry ice cream" for two days. Two days prior to admission he had eaten a bowl of cereal, the components of which were coated with Red No. 2 and Red No. 3. All blood studies and the physical examination of the youngster were normal, and his stools returned to normal color. When given another bowl of the cereal, his stools again turned red. A sibling was also noted to have this same problem. This appears to be a harmless but rather spectacular episode in the saga of the food dyes.

Trichloroethylene

As mentioned in Chapter 3, the National Cancer Institute in 1975 issued a "Memorandum of Alert" concerning the chemical trichloroethylene. Studies at the NCI revealed that the chemical, when fed in large quantities to mice, caused liver and other cancers to develop.

It so happens that trichloroethylene is used in the food processing industry to remove caffeine from coffee. Current government standards allow trace amounts of the chemical to remain in the finished product. Sanka and Brim, manufactured by General Foods, are both processed in this manner.

Dr. Sidney Wolfe, director of the Health Research Group, stated that continued use of the chemical should be banned and that the situation is an "open and shut violation of the Delaney Clause which prohibits the presence of known carcinogens in the food supply." Wolfe pointed out that the trace amounts of trichloroethylene can be ingested when the decaffeinated coffee is consumed and can even be inhaled in fumes from the coffee cup. Subsequently, General Foods discontinued the use of TCE and substituted the chemical methylene chloride for use in the decaffeination process. Methylene chloride is a chemical which has not been tested for cancer-producing properties.

In June, 1976, the National Cancer Institute issued a final report on the bioassay of TCE. The report concluded that the chemical clearly induced liver cancer in mice, and the findings should serve as a warning of possible carcinogenicity in humans. At the same time, the National Cancer Institute issued a statement on substitution of chemicals not tested for carcinogenicity. In this statement, the institute expressed its concern that before replacing a chemical found to be carcinogenic in a bioassay, the alternative compounds should also be evaluated adequately in terms of carcinogenicity. Otherwise, the replacement of a chemical having a certain estimated risk with another chemical of unknown risk may mean the adoption of a more hazardous alternative.

Monosodium Glutamate

So far we have discussed foods and food additives that may be carcinogenic, cause birth defects, or cause mutations—

processes that may take years to become manifest. Let's now turn our attention to chemicals in foods that manifest their toxicity more rapidly. First let's look at monosodium glutamate, abbreviated MSG. There has been much controversy about this chemical, which is used extensively in Chinese food as a flavor enhancer. It is also added to commercially prepared baby foods for the same purpose.

A syndrome called "Kwok's quease" has been reported among patrons of Chinese restaurants. This syndrome consists of several neurological symptoms and has been attributed to a high intake of MSG in the food. Experimental studies of MSG are numerous. Very high doses administered to young chickens are fatal. Infant mice developed brain lesions following administration of MSG. Similar findings have been noted in rats. However, in another study, monkeys given varying doses of the chemical and killed six hours after treatment had no brain changes. In general, lower levels of MSG did not produce anatomical verification of the symptoms of "Kwok's quease."

Biochemical studies are more enlightening. A study of the enzyme systems in the livers and brains of mice given MSG showed that the chemical interfered with the uptake of sugar by brain tissue, and the response was dose-related. This offers a plausible explanation for the symptoms of "Kwok's quease." Additional studies have supported this relationship. Experiments designed to detect possible behavioral abnormalities in rats treated neonatally with MSG definitely showed lower discrimination aptitude in all dose ranges tested. Rats receiving high doses of MSG also showed decreased spontaneous motor activity. Maze learning capacity was depressed at all dose levels.

MSG finally was removed from baby food in 1969 after nutritionists and consumer protection groups charged that the chemical was needless and dangerous to infants' nervous systems. It was stated that MSG had no nutritional value and that it was added to conceal the overuse of starches and the underuse of meats.

Sodium Bisulphite

Another additive that scientists are having second thoughts about is the preservative sodium bisulphite. It is used in numerous foods, including canned potato chips. In addition to its preservative effects, sodium bisulphite also improves the color of food and drinks. Until recently, it was thought that the only detrimental effect of the sulphites was to inactivate the vitamin thiamine. However, it has been discovered that sodium bisulphite also interferes with nucleic acid synthesis.

More sophisticated studies need to be performed to determine the safety of this chemical. One recent study demonstrated that rats fed sodium bisulphite (2 percent) up to two years and over three generations displayed slight retardation in the second and third generations. Mild gastrointestinal bleeding was noted in groups given 1 percent or more. Hyperplastic changes were noted in the stomach lining of all groups fed 1 percent or 2 percent. There was no indication of any carcinogenic effect. Higher dosages caused considerable growth depression. Enlarged spleens were noted with 4 percent or more in the diet. Stomach ulcers occurred at 6 percent and 8 percent dosage levels. Low levels of sulphite (0.25 percent) had no untoward effects in rats.

Several scientists have warned of the possibility that sodium bisulphite may cause mutations.

Carrageenan

Carrageenan is another additive widely used in the food and toiletry industries as a jelling agent. It is found in chocolate milk, milk puddings, water-gel desserts, and commercial infant formulas (Similac, Enfamil), and it is used to thicken soups, sauces, and gravies. It is a sulfated polygalactoside obtained from seaweeds. In 1970 the Joint FAO/WHO Expert Committee on Food Additives recommended limiting daily intake to 50 milligrams per kilogram in man. Since that time, scientists have reported lesions resembling ulcerative colitis in rats, guinea pigs, and rabbits fed carrageenan. Monkeys fed the degraded form of carrageenan lost blood from the intestinal tract and had ulcerative lesions. The severity of the symptoms was related to the dose.

The degraded form of carrageenan has a molecular weight of around 30,000. Extract derived from the seaweed is called native carrageenan and has a molecular weight of 100,000 to 800,000. This is the form used as a food additive. In mild acid solution, carrageenan is broken into the degraded form. Studies in monkeys have shown that native carrageenan does not cause any discernible effect. However, administration of the degraded form led to intestinal blood loss and anemia.

Recently, carrageenan has become suspect for another reason. Food and Drug Administration tests of the chemical have produced liver lesions in laboratory rats. In light of these findings, common sense dictates that one not eat foods containing carrageenan. The magazine *Consumer Reports* (March 1975) reviewed the carrageenan problem and also recommended that even though the FDA had not taken official steps to halt the use of carrageenan, consumers should avoid this food additive until its safety can be determined. The magazine pointed out that consumers can identify products containing carrageenan by reading the labels on the food containers.

Antioxidants (BHT and BHA)

Another group of commonly used food additives are the antioxidants. Although suspicion was cast on their safety several years ago, scientists now believe that this group of additives may also have some beneficial side effects. The most widely used of these is butylated hydroxytoluene, or BHT. It is found in most packaging materials for cereals, mixes, and other dry packaged foods. Antioxidants are added to both human and animal food as preservatives for unsaturated fats and other food components subject to spoilage by oxidation.

These compounds produce a variety of physiological effects in animals, including a reduction in growth rate, elevated serum cholesterol, and liver changes, including liver enlargement and increased enzymatic activity. On the other hand, several antioxidants have been reported to increase the lifespan of mice. The antioxidant BHT was found to reduce the incidence of tumors produced by certain carcinogens but not by others. In another study another commonly used antioxidant, BHA, inhibited tumor formation in a similar manner. While some investigators attribute this supression of carcinogenicity of certain chemicals to the antioxidant properties of these agents, others disagree.

At the present time the reason for the effect remains obscure.

The authors of the cited BHT study are internationally recognized experts in chemical carcinogenesis and state that the data available from the sizable studies on antioxidants in animal model systems more often than not demonstrated a decrease in carcinogenic effects of known carcinogens. They also state that these agents are similar in structure and physiological properties to vitamin E. They contend that in the light of the potentially beneficial effect of these agents, the current attitude toward the use of these agents in foods needs to be reexamined.

5
Consumer
Products

Each year thousands of new products are introduced to the consumer market. Many of these products contain chemicals that come in contact with the consumer in a variety of ways. Strict regulations and standards for these products in terms of exposure of the consumer to potential carcinogens do not exist at the present writing. Unwitting or unscrupulous manufacturers are at liberty to market these products without prior testing. Scientists regard many products as "suspicious"—such items as flame-retardant clothes and formaldehyde-containing holding tank disinfectant that may possibly form the highly carcinogenic bis (chloromethyl) ether during normal consumer use, asbestos-containing products, and vinyl chloride-containing products, just to name a few. Literally hundreds of other products also are in the "suspicious" category.

Again, the problem is our own ignorance. The appropriate tests have not been performed on these products, nor are they required, and we play Russian roulette every time a new product is released in the marketplace. The solution is the establishment of a tough consumer protection agency that would require every manufacturer to submit proof that its new product is harmless. There is much pressure from industry against this sort of legislation because the testing is both expensive and time-consuming. Furthermore, the product may be proved harmful and marketing would be prohibited.

Such a consumer protection agency was to have been formed, but it was vetoed by President Nixon as one of his final acts as President. It may turn out to be one of his greatest mistakes.

Two consumer products in particular have been shown by epidemiologic studies to be responsible for large numbers of human cancers. These products are so much a part of our way of life that it will be very difficult to stop or even limit their use. They sustain two of our more popular vices—smoking and drinking. For those of you who now say at least we have sex left, if you are female, don't count on it! Studies strongly suggest that if a female begins sexual relations at an early age with multiple partners, her chances of getting cancer of the cervix are much higher than if she started later and with fewer partners. From all this information, we must now change the adage that "anything I like is either illegal, immoral, or fattening" to "anything I like is either illegal, immoral, fattening, or causes cancer."

Tobacco

It has been estimated that tobacco use kills about 360,000 people annually in the United States. A wide range of maladies has been directly linked with smoking, including chronic obstructive pulmonary disease, emphysema, and lung cancer and other malignancies. The surgeon general's first report on smoking, linking the habit with the diseases cited, was published in January 1964, yet cigarette smoking continues at an all-time high. In 1975 over 660 billion U.S.-made cigarettes were expected to go up in smoke. This leads one to conclude that either people are very stupid or cigarette smoking is a very difficult habit to break.

The economic loss from cigarette smoking is staggering. Many smokers could buy a luxury automobile with the money they have spent for cigarettes. The time lost from productive work due to nonmalignant respiratory disease is phenomenal. Respiratory diseases caused by smoking include benign maladies such as upper respiratory infections and increases in severity to bronchitis, pneumonia, and finally disabling chronic obstructive pulmonary disease and pulmonary emphysema, which leaves the smoker a permanent respiratory cripple, gasping for breath—a rather uncomfortable situation. Needless to say, hospital and doctor bills add considerably to the cost.

In addition to the nonmalignant respiratory diseases, heart attacks and blood vessel diseases are more frequent among smokers.

Infants born to smoking mothers also are adversely affected. Smoking mothers have a greater number of unsuccessful pregnancies due to stillbirth and neonatal death, and the smoker has nearly twice the risk of delivering a low-birth-weight infant than the nonsmoker. If smoking impairs the fetus to this extent, one must wonder whether there will be long-term effects that will manifest themselves later in life. Will the carcinogens in cigarette smoke make the baby of a smoking mother more susceptible to cancer later in life than a child born to a nonsmoking mother? There is some evidence to support this suspicion. Carcinogens in cigarette smoke inhaled by the mother during pregnancy have been shown to cross the placenta and enter the fetus.

The relationship between cancer and smoking has been well established by a number of studies. Not only is lung cancer related to smoking, but malignancies of the lips, tongue, throat, larnyx, esophagus, and bladder are as well—and all are unpleasant fates.

A 1972 study of the relative risk of oral cancer according to smoking habits revealed that if one smoked less than forty cigarettes per day, he was one and one-half times more likely to get oral cancer than if he did not smoke at all. If one smoked forty or more cigarettes per day, his chances were two and one-half times greater than if he did not smoke.

The heavy use of cigarettes in the early teen-age years is responsible for an alarming incidence of bladder cancer among men in their late twenties through early fifties. If diagnosed early, these tumors are usually curable if they are surgically removed and if the patient stops smoking. If he continues to smoke, the tumor is likely to recur.

Both chemical carcinogens and co-carcinogens have been isolated from cigarette smoke. Today's cigarettes yield less tar and nicotine than their counterparts of twenty years ago, and they produce fewer tumors in experimental animals. These "safer cigarettes" should result in lowering the incidence of cancer among smokers, but how much the rate will be lowered remains to be seen. Obviously, the nonsmoker is still safer than the smoker.

Many smokers have given up the habit, with highly educated males far in the lead. Antismoking campaigns have been less effective among young people because of peer group pressure equating smoking with adulthood. Boys have maintained their rate of taking up smoking, while girls have increased their rate to equal that of boys.

Considering the gravity of the situation, very little has been done to reduce smoking since the surgeon general's report was published twelve years ago. We must raise the question why society, government, and the scientific community have not done more to combat this one factor that is responsible for so much disability, economic loss, and human suffering.

There is some suggestion that smoking may affect one's sex life. Many people who quit smoking notice an improvement in their sexual desires and performance soon afterward. Studies have shown a greater decline in sexual activity with age among smokers as opposed to nonsmokers. Several physiological factors tend to substantiate this finding. Smoking hampers pulmonary function and stamina, and smokers tire more easily than non-smokers. Smoking hastens vascular disease and aging processes. Furthermore, smoking reduces sexual attractiveness by causing foul breath and discolored teeth. Perhaps this interference with one's sex life will be more of a deterrent to smoking than threat of cancer and lung disease.

Alcohol

The effects of alcohol on society are monumental. An estimated two million persons in the United States alone are alcoholics. No other chemical affects so large a population with such devastating results in terms of human misery, economic loss, and waste of life. What other over-the-counter chemical is able to turn a rational human being into a slobbering idiot? But enough said about the effects of alcohol on society. That is outside the scope of this book.

What is within the scope of this book are the long-term chronic effects of alcohol on human health. Much can be said about that subject.

According to epidemiologic studies, excessive alcohol consumption increases the risk of cancer in several organs. There is good evidence to link alcoholism with tumors of the head, neck, esophagus, and liver. There is also some evidence suggesting a link between alcohol and cancer of the pancreas and prostate gland. As one might expect, these studies showed that the higher the intake and the longer the duration of intake, the greater the risk for developing cancer.

Based on its molecular structure and metabolism, alcohol appears unlikely to be a carcinogen. In fact, mice raised on a regimen of 20 percent alcohol in their drinking water did not develop tumors even after prolonged exposure. However, alcohol appears to enhance the action of known carcinogens in the production of tumors. This has been demonstrated with the carcinogen DMBA (dimethyl benz-(a)-anthracene) in the production of tumors of the mouth and skin. Studies such as this suggest that alcohol acts as a co-carcinogen with other carcinogens to which we are exposed. Most alcoholic beverages themselves contain small amounts of suspected or known carcinogens in addition to the alcohol.

Approximately one of every 300 heavy drinkers will develop cancer of the mouth, tongue, or throat. According to one study this incidence is almost six times greater than expected among nondrinkers. In another study intake of less than 0.4 ounces of alcohol per day increased the chance of developing oral cancer by 40 percent, and the incidence increased with higher daily intake. This study also showed that smoking increased the risk of oral cancer considerably, and if one were both a heavy smoker and drank more than one and one-half ounces of alcohol per day, his chance of developing oral cancer skyrocketed to fifteen times greater than that of the nonsmoker and nondrinker. Consumption of hard liquor is more likely to cause these tumors than is beer or wine. There is also a strong association between tumors of the mouth and throat and cirrhosis of the liver.

Cancer of the larynx is also associated with alcoholism, and as with mouth and throat tumors, whiskey is more likely to produce laryngeal tumors than is beer or wine. Unfortunately, these tumors are often diagnosed late in the course of the disease in alcoholics because the early symptoms of hoarseness and voice change are often overlooked in the heavy drinker.

A definite association has been established between cancer of the esophagus and alcoholism. The disease appears to be increasing in the United States, especially in the nonwhite urban population. The esophagus is the first portion of the digestive system to be exposed to alcoholic beverages. The type of beverage consumed and the particular form of carbohydrate used in its preparation appears to be related to the production of these tumors, probably due to different carcinogens formed in the brewing process. In France the highest incidence of esophageal cancer is found in areas where the main alcoholic beverage is apple brandy, rather than wine. In parts of eastern and southern Africa, cancer of the esophagus is almost epidemic, and it appears that the disease is seen more frequently where beer is produced from fermented maize rather than from bananas, millet, or honey. In Puerto Rico, home-processed rum is thought to be responsible for the high incidence of the disease.

The incidence of liver cancer varies widely geographically. The higher incidence in certain parts of the world is thought to be related to the consumption of aflatoxins. However, in North America and Europe, liver cancer is most likely to occur in people with alcoholic cirrhosis of the liver. The percentage of people with alcoholic cirrhosis of the liver who develop liver cancer has been reported to range from 8 percent to as high as 30 percent. Cirrhosis of the liver produced by causes other than alcohol appear to pose less risk of developing into cancer than do the alcohol-induced variety.

The pancreas is second only to the liver in vulnerability to the effects of alcohol. Both acute and chronic pancreatitis are caused by alcohol, and there is now some question whether cancer of the pancreas is related to alcohol ingestion as well. Many patients who die of pancreatic cancer have had pancreatitis, but this may be due in part to effects of the cancer itself. Epidemiologic studies have shown a significantly greater incidence of alcoholism in a group of patients who died from cancer of the pancreas than in a comparable control group dying from other causes. Other studies suggest a positive relationship between alcohol and pancreatic cancer, but it still cannot be said with absolute certainty that the relationship does exist. Further studies are needed.

There is also some evidence to suggest an association between cancer of the prostate gland and alcohol. A study of alcoholics in Norway revealed a higher than expected incidence of the disease. Two other studies of the causes of death among alcoholics have also suggested this relationship.

There now appears to be little doubt that chronic ingestion of alcohol predisposes us to several types of cancer.

Another unfortunate effect of chronic alcoholism has been reported in medical literature recently. The "fetal alcohol syndrome" is a series of abnormalities occurring in the children of female alcoholics. The specific pattern involves prenatal growth deficiency, developmental delay, craniofacial anomalies, and limb defects. One or more of these defects or other adverse effects are seen in 43 percent of pregnancies in chronic alcoholic women.

The association between maternal alcoholism and serious problems in the offspring is not a new observation. Classical Greek and Roman mythology suggested that maternal alcoholism at the time of conception could lead to serious problems in fetal development, and this led to an ancient Carthaginian rule forbidding the drinking of wine by a bridal couple on their wedding night so that defective children would not be conceived.

A 1967 study of 127 children born to alcoholic parents revealed a frequent incidence of growth deficiency beginning in the prenatal period, unusual facial appearance, and a 25 percent incidence of birth defects, especially cleft palate and heart malformations. Mental retardation, "agitation," and character disturbances were frequently noted.

An autopsy on a child who died from fetal alcohol syndrome revealed extensive brain malformation, which probably accounts for the mental retardation and other brain-related symptoms seen in these children.

Another study of the outcome of twenty-three pregnancies among women who were chronic alcoholics compared the offspring of the alcoholics to socioeconomically paired control offspring of nonalcoholic mothers. The results were striking, pointing out the magnitude of the handicapping problems that alcoholism can impose on the developing fetus. Four of the twenty-three offspring of women who were alcoholics before and during pregnancy died before one week of age. This is a perinatal mortality rate of 17 percent as opposed to a rate of only 2 percent for offspring of nonalcoholic mothers. The surviving children had a high incidence of the symptoms of the fetal alcohol syndrome, and in the final analysis, 43 percent of these offspring suffered adverse effects as opposed to 2 percent for the controls.

The cancer-producing effects of smoking and drinking are well supported by epidemiologic and laboratory studies. Two other widely used consumer products have recently been regarded with a high degree of suspicion. They are food packaging materials and aerosol sprays.

Packaging Materials

It has been estimated that about 150 million pounds of vinyl chloride are used for food packaging annually. The PVC food packaging materials include plastic bottles, "blister" packs used for bologna and other sandwich meats, and other semirigid and rigid packaging. It is used in pliable film-type wraps (used to wrap meat in the supermarket), gaskets, cap liners, tubing and package coatings that come in contact with food, including coatings inside beer and soft drink cans. PVC also is used in coatings applied to fresh citrus fruits to retain freshness.

All plastic packaging materials contain a number of additives from their manufacture. These additives include plasticizers, stabilizers, pigments, accelerators, and other chemicals. Migration of both the plastic monomer and the plasticizers into the food they are supposed to protect is known to occur. Temperature, the type of plastic material, the nature of the food being contained, and the duration of contact between the two influence the quantity of additives and parent plastic monomer migrating into the food. The long-term toxicity of plasticizers in humans is unknown.

Tests have shown that the greatest amount of migration of vinyl chloride into food occurs in PVC bottles and semirigid packages. The problem has been recognized by the Food and Drug Administration. In 1973 the FDA banned the use of PVC liquor bottles after it was discovered that vinyl chloride was migrating into the liquor. In the summer of 1975 the FDA proposed a ban on the use of PVC containers of the bottle and semirigid type, as well as fruit sprays, but would allow the continued use of the PVC film wrap, cap liners, gaskets, and coatings in beer and soft drink cans on the basis that the migration of vinyl chloride is lower in these products. This proposal is still being considered at this writing.

Consumer groups have been pushing the FDA for a total ban on the use of PVC in food packaging. Industry is arguing, on the other hand, that the trace amounts of vinyl chloride found in foods are not sufficient to cause health concerns, and improved production processes are reducing the amount of vinyl chloride migration from plastic containers. (During production, some of the vinyl chloride gas is trapped in the solid plastic and is leached out by certain foods, particularly alcohols and fatty substances.) The FDA maintains that tests show that vinyl chloride migration is not a problem with the forms of packaging still allowed by the proposed ban.

Unfortunately, inadequate consideration has been given to the amounts of plasticizer migrating into our foods. Although the migration of vinyl chloride from film wrap is minimal, migration of plasticizer from other plastic containers is considerable with certain foods, and long-term toxicity data on plasticizers are lacking.

Polyvinyl chloride is also used extensively for packaging products for medicinal uses, including blood bags, bags for IV fluids, IV tubing, and other purposes. Pure PVC is actually a rigid substance, and the addition of plasticizers during the manufacturing process makes the stiff plastic more supple. One commonly used plasticizer, di(2-ethylhexyl) phthalate (DEHP) is extracted from PVC bags and tubing by blood products and IV fluids, and this has caused considerable concern in certain clinical situations. Deaths from intestinal perforation have occurred in newborn infants due to the accumulation of plasticizers from PVC bags and IV tubing used during exchange transfusions. The plasticizers appear to affect the blood vessels in the intestine, causing an interruption in the blood supply with subsequent death of the affected portion.

Other chemicals used in the food packaging industry have not been tested for carcinogenicity, mutagenicity, or teratogenicity and must also be regarded with some suspicion because of their chemical structures. These include other plastics, waxes, and other agents used for waterproofing, heat-treating, and strengthening purposes.

Aerosol Spray Cans

Has it ever occurred to you that the next time you spray a bug with insect killer, you may not only be rapidly killing the bug, but be slowly killing yourself as well? Who would ever think that such a useful invention could some day destroy all life on earth? Incredible as it sounds, this may be possible. Highly respected scientists are extremely concerned about the aerosol spray can—not the can itself, of course, but what is in it.

Let's look at the history of the spray can. The modern aerosol spray can was developed in the early 1950s following two discoveries. Chemists at the E. I. duPont de Nemours & Company found that a mixture of two gases, trichloromonofluoromethane and dichlorodifluoromethane, made an ideal propellant. They could be confined under low pressure in tin-plate or aluminum cans. Both gases had been synthesized in 1928 by research chemists in the General Motors research laboratories in an attempt to discover a new refrigerant. One of the gases, dichlorodifluoromethane, has been used widely since then as a coolant in refrigerators and air conditioners. Both gases are manufactured now by the duPont Company under the trade name of Freon. Both gases are chemically "inert" and do not react with the products or ingredients in spray cans.

The second important discovery leading to the development

of the aerosol spray can was the invention of the mass-producible dispensing valve by Robert H. Abplanalb.

By 1954 the annual production of aerosol spray cans was 188 million, most of them dispensing insecticides and shaving cream. By 1958 production soared to over 500 million cans, with hair-sprays taking over as the leading item. By 1968 the annual production topped two billion cans.

By 1970 aerosol cans had more than 300 different uses—dispensing such products as oven cleaner, breath sweeteners, weed killers, cheese spreads, rug shampoo, and whipped-cream substitutes. Today, aerosols are a $3-billion-a-year industry. In 1973, 2,900,340,000 aerosol spray cans were manufactured in the United States alone. In 1974 the figure topped four billion, about 50 percent of the total world production. It is estimated that the average American family has at least forty aerosol spray cans in various parts of the house.

There was not much concern about the tremendous production and release of propellant gases into the environment until 1974, when scientists discovered that these gases might be threatening the environment. The first suggestion that this might be the case was noted in 1970, when Dr. James E. Lovelock, an English biospheric chemist at the University of Reading, detected one of the propellant gases, trichloromonofluoromethane, in the air over western Ireland. He assumed that the other gas, dichlorodifluoromethane, also was present. His assumption was later confirmed.

In 1971 Lovelock subsequently measured air samples over the Atlantic Ocean and found trichloromonofluoromethane in the troposphere—the six-to-ten-mile-high portion of the atmosphere. Lovelock and other scientists at first regarded the ubiquitous presence of the chemicals as harmless.

Upon hearing of Lovelock's discovery that the chlorofluorocarbons were present throughout the troposphere, Dr. F. Sherwood Rowland, a chemist at the University of California, began to wonder where the chemicals were going and what would become of them. Rowland was a specialist in the chemistry of radioactive isotopes. On October 1, 1973, he and Dr. Mario J. Molina, a photochemist who had recently joined Rowland's research staff, began to study the problem. They knew that the chlorofluorocarbons could be decomposed upon photolysis by short-wavelength ultraviolet light from the sun, and that this decomposition would have to occur high in the stratosphere because almost all short-wavelength ultraviolet light from the sun is filtered out of the lower levels by the ozone layer. They knew that the chlorofluorocarbons, being stable compounds, would survive long enough to rise eventually to these high levels of the stratosphere where the chemical decomposition could take place. They estimated that if the production of these compounds continued at the 1972 worldwide rate of almost one million tons a year, the several million tons now in the troposphere would increase dramatically.

In November 1973 Rowland and Molina studied the inevitable reaction between the chlorofluorocarbons and ultraviolet light. Their findings were disturbing. When chlorine was released from the breakdown of the chlorofluorocarbons, it reacted with a molecule of ozone, which in turn initiated an extensive and catalytic chain reaction that decomposed as many as a hundred thousand molecules of ozone. The finding that a single atom of chlorine could cause the destruction of such large quantities of ozone was disturbing.

They recalled from their earlier calculations that nearly one hundred million tons of chlorofluorocarbons could be expected to build up in the troposphere in the next century or so, and enough chlorine would be produced roughly to double the depletion of ozone known to occur naturally each year. Further calculations led them to estimate that eventually from 20 to 40 percent of the ozone could be destroyed. This would cause a tremendous increase in the kind of solar radiation known to be detrimental to both plant and animal life. They calculated that if the production of the chlorofluorocarbons continued to increase at the present rate of 10 percent per year until 1990 and remained constant after that, between 5 and 7 percent of the ozone layer would be destroyed by 1995, and from 30 to 50 percent would be destroyed by the year 2050. They went on to warn that partial destruction of the ozone layer would, because of the increase in ultraviolet radiation to the surface of the earth, cause a large increase in the incidence of skin cancer, and as the radiation increased with accelerated destruction of the ozone layer, other more serious biological effects would result, including genetic mutations and crop damage. Changes in world weather patterns might also occur, and the problem would be irreversible. They pointed out that if nothing were done in the next decade to prevent the further release of the chemicals, continuing destruction of the ozone layer would occur for most of the twenty-first century. In their report to the American Chemical Society in September 1974, they stated that in their opinion, the advantage of using chlorofluorocarbons as propellants and refrigerants was not worth the risks they posed to the environment, and they urged that the use of these compounds be banned.

The aerosol industry countered these charges by pointing out that the calculations of Rowland and Molina were hypothetical and that no real proof existed that the two gases could rise into the stratosphere, much less cause the destruction of ozone. Dr. Raymond McCarthy, technical director of duPont's Freon products division, announced that a three-year industry-sponsored study of the problem would begin. He stated that it would be an injustice if hypothesis alone were to serve as a basis for judgment and action against the use of these chemicals.

The furor led to a congressional inquiry. On December 11, 1974, the Subcommittee on Public Health and Environment of the House Committee on Interstate and Foreign Commerce began two days of hearings to consider regulating or banning the manufacture of the chlorofluorocarbons. No action was taken because the Ninety-third Congress expired eight days after the hearings were concluded.

In February 1975 two bills were introduced into the House of Representatives regarding the problem, but both bills avoided banning the gases. They called for additional studies to be performed to determine whether a chain reaction initiated by chlorine released from the gases is in fact destroying the ozone layer. The studies were to be performed by the National Academy of Sciences and the National Aeronautics and Space Administration and were scheduled to be completed by spring 1976.

There is evidence that aerosol sprays are more immediately hazardous to the millions of people who have been inhaling them. Freons themselves are known to cause death from cardiac arrest when inhaled at high concentrations, and medical literature reports deaths of patients while using spray cans. In addition to breathing the propellant gases from spray cans, there is the additional danger of breathing the aerosolized product—the hairspray, deodorant, paint, cleaner, and so on. Aerosolization causes the formation of very small droplets of the chemical, which can be breathed into the lungs of the user. This provides an access route for the chemical into the body—into the bloodstream and all the organs. Prior to the use of aerosol spray cans these chemicals did not have access to our innards. Now we are exposing ourselves to thousands of new chemicals, some of which are highly suspicious on the basis of chemical structure but have never been tested for a variety of possible toxic effects, including cancer, mutations, birth defects, and organ damage.

The plastic resins used in hairsprays are suspected of causing both restrictive lung disease and changes in lung cells that may lead to cancer. A study by Dr. Alan Palmer, an epidemiologist with the National Institute for Occupational Safety and Health, found that nearly 50 percent of 500 cosmetologists had symptoms of early obstructive lung disease, such as asthma and emphysema.

Even more disturbing was the finding in 1974 that vinyl chloride, used as the propellant in many aerosol products, is a human carcinogen. Upon learning this, the Japanese government spent $25 million to impound all aerosols containing the chemical. However, our government agencies, which are supposed to protect the public, did little more than request the aerosol-producing companies to stop using vinyl chloride as a propellant. As a result, millions of spray cans containing vinyl chloride stayed on store shelves and in homes. The consumer had no way of telling which cans contained the cancer-causing agent. It is listed on the can as an "inert ingredient." Studies have shown that use of a vinyl chloride–propelled spray can under normal conditions, such as a woman spraying her hair in a small room, can contaminate the room with up to 250 parts per million of vinyl chloride. Since it is known that as low as 50 ppm of vinyl chloride can produce cancer in rats, the Department of Labor's Occupational Safety and Health Administration has set the upper limit of safety for industrial workers at 1 ppm. The hairspray may produce up to 250 times this level, yet our government agencies did little to protect us from the products that were already in circulation.

There is a valuable lesson to learn from the aerosol sprays. That lesson is the necessity of testing potentially harmful substances before they are allowed on the market. This is necessary for the protection of the consumer, the worker, and the environment.

Pesticides

A book about the causes of cancer would not be complete without a section on pesticides. Several pesticides have now been shown to produce cancer in various laboratory animals. This fact, together with the known world wide distribution of these chemicals—even in remote areas—is cause for great concern.

The best-known insecticide is DDT, or dichlorodiphenyl-trichloroethane. It is a white, crystalline, water-insoluble solid that is fairly stable, so it remains in the environment for a long time. DDT may accumulate in large amounts. It has been found in agricultural soils at concentrations as high as one hundred pounds per acre!

DDT, like other long-lasting pesticides, accumulates in food chains. Such pesticides are concentrated as they pass up the chain so that predators at the top of the chain are often severely affected. For example, earthworms are fairly resistant to DDT and may accumulate a fair amount of the chemical without dying. But about one hundred of the contaminated worms may be fatal to a robin. Furthermore, DDT affects calcium metabolism in birds so that their eggshells become fragile and break prior to hatching. Because of this problem, certain avian species, including the peregrine falcon, the bald eagle, and the gannet, are in danger of extinction.

It is not surprising that DDT and other pesticides have been found in human tissue. In the United States in the late 1960s the body tissues of the "average" person contained up to 12 parts per million DDT, and detectable levels were present in human milk. Except for people with occupational exposure to DDT, the major source of exposure is residues in foods. An analysis of typical meals served in the United Kingdom in 1965 revealed an average daily intake of 0.02 milligrams DDT. The insecticide dieldrin was consumed at an average of 0.06 milligrams per day. The high fat solubility of these chlorinated hydrocarbon insecticides is responsible for their uptake and storage in fatty tissue. An English study of 101 autopsies in 1965 showed an average of 2.23 ppm DDT and 0.23 ppm dieldrin in human fat.

In another study autopsy specimens of human fat from residents of Dade County (Miami), Florida, were analyzed for pesticide concentrations. The residents were classified as to whether they used pesticides (1) sparingly, or not at all, (2) moderately, or (3) with little regard for safety. DDT levels in thirty-one residents who used pesticides sparingly (in home or garden only) averaged 9.4 ppm. Sixty-five moderate users averaged 19.4 ppm, and twenty-two users with little regard for safety averaged 27 ppm. This study showed that we can do much to protect ourselves by keeping our exposure at a minimum. None of the users cited was occupationally exposed to pesticides. The first group, those who used pesticides sparingly or not at all, probably represents a baseline level of intake due mainly·to the ingestion of pesticide residues in foods.

As expected, those with occupational exposure to pesticides have considerably higher levels than the general population. A study of thirty-five workers exposed to DDT for eleven to nineteen years had levels ranging from 38 to 647 ppm in their body fat.

The tumor-producing properties of DDT were first suspected as early as 1947 when a commercial preparation of the chemical was fed to rats, providing up to 800 ppm in the diet over a period of two years. The study revealed that DDT did indeed have minimal tendencies to cause the formation of liver tumors after eighteen months of feeding. In 1967 scientists fed 75 ppm DDT to rainbow trout. After fifteen months, liver tumors were found in seven of nineteen fish, and after twenty months, in four of eleven fish. Three hundred control fish that did not ingest DDT had only two liver tumors. Another study in 1969 revealed that mice fed DDT had a significant increase in the occurrence of both liver tumors and lymphomas.

Multigenerational studies with DDT, or studies of the

offspring of animals exposed to the chemical over several generations, produced interesting and rather disturbing results. The incidence of tumors and leukemias was studied in five mouse generations from original parents who were fed 3 ppm DDT in their diet. Twenty-six months after the study started, the youngest of the five generations was eleven months old. All animals were examined at that time. The overall tumor and leukemia incidence was 12.4 percent and 28.7 percent respectively, while the control group incidence was only 2.5 percent and 3.2 percent respectively. The proportions of tumors and leukemias did not appear to change with succeeding generations, yet the youngest generations had more tumors appearing earlier in life. Had the fourth and fifth generations been allowed to live as long as the earlier generations, they would probably have had an even higher incidence of malignancies. If further studies show this pattern to be true, and if the data are applicable to humans, it would suggest disaster for the human race. Fortunately, DDT was banned from general use as an insecticide in 1972.

The tumor-producing effects of pesticides from spray cans have recently been investigated. Freon propellants are the pressure source for most commercial pesticide spray cans. Scientists examined combinations of Freon 112 and Freon 113 and the insecticide piperonyl butoxide by injecting combinations of the chemicals into newborn mice. It was found that the combined chemicals produced a much greater incidence of liver tumors than did each chemical when injected alone.

Other pesticides, too, have been shown to be carcinogenic. In 1954 the fumigant β-propriolactone was shown to be a skin carcinogen when applied to rodents. It has not as yet been implicated as a human carcinogen. Another pesticide, bis (2-chloroethyl) ether, was shown to be a liver carcinogen in mice at the concentration of 300 ppm in the diet. Arsenic-containing pesticides are also regarded with great suspicion.

A pesticide that has recently come under fire is dieldrin. In 1974 the Environmental Protection Agency banned the use of dieldrin in the United States. This ban was the culmination of several years of bitter debate between scientists and environmentalists on the one hand and Shell Oil Company, the manufacturer, on the other. As early as March 1971 the EPA announced tentative plans to cancel the use of dieldrin. Shell appealed, and over the next several years the controversy raged, with more than 20,000 pages of testimony produced. In October 1974 the EPA suspended the use of dieldrin on grounds that it was an "imminent hazard" to human health.

About 10 percent of the dieldrin used in the United States has been for the eradication of termites. The remainder has been used as a prophylactic measure in growing corn. However, the major pest for this crop, the corn worm, is resistant to dieldrin. The continued use of this chemical would result in its becoming a major environmental contaminant. It has already reached measurable levels in New Orleans drinking water (70 parts per trillion) and has been measured in the fat of humans. Levels of dieldrin have surpassed the maximum tolerable limit in Lake Michigan fish, resulting in seizure of batches of commercially caught fish from that lake.

Dieldrin has been shown to produce cancer in five different strains of mice at doses as low as 0.1 parts per million. Several different types of tumors have been reported. Other experiments have produced tumors in rats.

Two other pesticides also have recently come under attack. During the summer of 1975 the EPA announced plans to suspend the use of chlordane and heptachlor because recent studies in rodents have implicated the chemicals as carcinogens. Both chlordane and heptachlor have chemical structures similar to those of other halogenated hydrocarbon insecticides such as dieldrin, lindane, and DDT (see Figure 1). Chlordane is one of the most widely used household and garden pesticides. Technical grade chlordane is actually a mixture of related compounds, the major one of which is chlordane itself. However, it also contains about 10 percent heptachlor.

Between 15 and 16 million pounds of chlordane were used in 1972—60 percent for termite control and other household uses. Both chlordane and heptachlor, or their metabolites, are persistent in the environment long after use. In market basket surveys, chlordane and related compounds were found commonly in dairy products, meat, fish, and poultry. Heptachlor compound residues

Figure 1
Chemical Structures of Some Commonly Used Insecticides

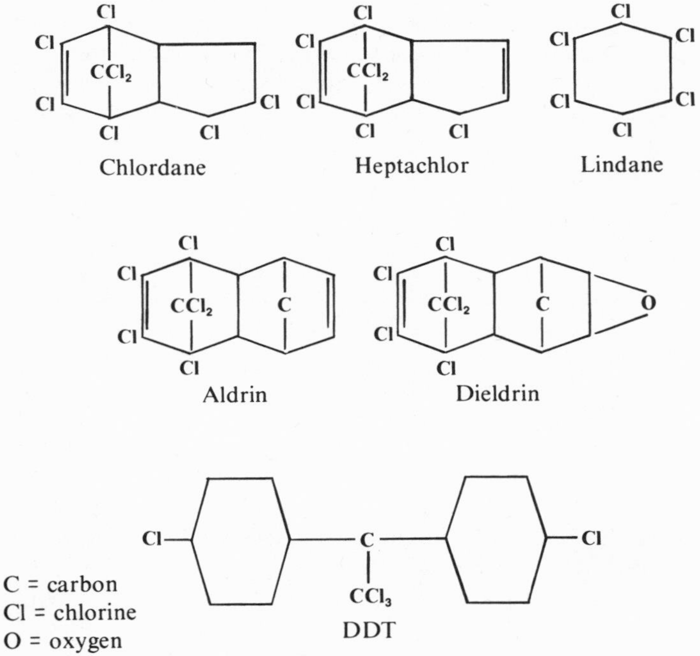

Chlordane   Heptachlor   Lindane

Aldrin   Dieldrin

C = carbon
Cl = chlorine
O = oxygen

DDT

have been detected in the organs of stillborn infants and also in samples of human milk, in fat samples of human adults, and in human fetuses.

The sole producer of both chlordane and heptachlor is Velsicol Chemical Corporation, a Chicago subsidiary of Northwest Industries. Velsicol produced about 21 million pounds of chlordane and 2 million pounds of heptachlor in 1974.

In December of 1975 EPA administrator Russell Train banned most uses of chlordane and heptachlor, including use of the pesticides on lawns, gardens, and turf and for household pest control. Train allowed the continued use of chlordane and heptachlor on some minor crops and against certain insects, including fire ants and termites.

Kepone, another insecticide that is used as an ant and roach poison, recently became both an occupational and environmental problem (see Chapter 3). Employees of the Life Science Products Company, Hopewell, Virginia, were hospitalized in 1975 with symptoms of Kepone poisoning—neurological symptoms, liver damage, and infertility. More than half of the company's employees were found to have relatively high levels of Kepone in their blood. The long-term effects of Kepone poisoning in humans are not known, but the chemical has been found to cause cancer in mice and rats. The Life Science plant was closed in July 1975 as a result of worker illness.

In December 1975 the Environmental Protection Agency announced that it had found traces of Kepone in the James River as far as forty miles from the Life Science production facility. Virginia Governor Mills E. Godwin subsequently closed the James River and its major tributaries to fishing.

What effect pesticides will have on the health of future human generations is unknown. Regulating agencies appear increasingly eager to curb the indiscriminate use of these chemicals. The major issue is the fact that trace amounts of pesticides enter our bodies from food, air, and water. We do not know how much pesticide intake can be tolerated without damage to health. The carcinogenic effects may be initiated at extremely low levels.

Formaldehyde

The chemical formaldehyde is used frequently in industry, and its industrial hazards are discussed in Chapter 3.

For the consumer, formaldehyde poses a serious threat to health because it can react with hydrochloric acid, which is present in human perspiration, urine, and vomitus, to form the potent cancer-causing chemical bis (chloromethyl) ether. Scientists are concerned that the formaldehyde residues present in childrens' flame-retardant and permanent-press clothes may react with these body fluids and expose the youngsters to BCME at a time in their lives when they are most susceptible to its carcinogenic effect.

Motor home owners will be interested to learn that several products on the market used to sanitize and deodorize mobile home toilet facilities contain formaldehyde. Scientists suspect that BCME may be formed every time someone uses the facilities in these vehicles. Not all products used for this purpose contain formaldehyde. The labels on the packages usually list the ingredients, so choose accordingly.

Numerous other consumer products could be discussed— hair dyes, cough remedies, auto rustproofing materials, and so on. The problem of dangerous consumer products is monumental. As suggested earlier, at least part of the answer lies in the formation of a consumer protection agency that would require mandatory testing of all new products and of all current products that are regarded as suspicious.

6
Water, Water, Everywhere

"Water, water, everywhere,
Nor any drop to drink."
—"The Rime of the Ancient Mariner,"
Samuel Taylor Coleridge

The quotation above expresses the predicament of a group on a ship becalmed at sea. The water—salt water—was poison to them.

If you are a city dweller in a large metropolitan area that derives its drinking water from a major river downstream from industrial plants, you may be in the same boat!

The problem was brought to the attention of the public on television and in the press in late 1974, but the information has been of concern to scientists for several years.

Industrial wastes, domestic sewage, and agricultural runoffs are pouring into our rivers and lakes in frightening quantities. Although municipal waters are treated primarily to make them microbiologically safe to drink, nothing is being done to remove—or better yet, prevent—the trace amounts of organic chemicals that enter our drinking water supplies.

Let's look at the water treatment system of a typical large city in the United States—Detroit. The system is a mammoth operation in terms of volume. Between 700 million and one billion gallons of water are pumped each day from the Detroit River and Lake Huron to be processed and then supplied to ninety-six communities, including Detroit. This system supplies water to four million people, about 45 percent of the population of Michigan.

Between the river and the household tap, the water is subjected to a series of purification procedures. It is first screened to remove fish and debris. Then chlorine is added to kill bacteria and microorganisms. Fluoride is then added. Next, the water is treated with aluminum sulfate and powered charcoal to remove suspended impurities and some chemicals that may affect its taste. During this process the water is also filtered through beds of sand and gravel. Finally, more chlorine is added.

Chlorination is the most important process, because it kills bacteria that would otherwise cause outbreaks of such diseases as typhoid, cholera, and dysentery. But now there is evidence that chlorine may react with certain chemical contaminants already present in the water to form chlorinated hydrocarbons, some of which are known to cause cancer.

Even though the water had not yet been checked for carcinogens, an official of the Detroit Water Department told the *Detroit Free Press* in April 1975 that Detroit's water was "about the purest in the country." At the same time he admitted that there may be some organic chemicals in the water from petroleum refineries up the Detroit River and in Sarnia, Ontario, and also some pesticide residues from the Great Lakes. He said that these chemicals are present in amounts too small to create a health hazard.

Many scientists disagree with the principles of this statement. One noted expert on chemical carcinogens, Dr. Samuel Epstein, recently testified before the Louisiana House Committee on Health and Welfare, saying "prudent public health policy demands that any chemical agent found after appropriate testing to be carcinogenic in one or more animal species should also be presumed to be carcinogenic in man in the absence of any evidence to the contrary."

Many experts in chemical carcinogenesis agree with Epstein, who also told the Louisiana legislators that the only "safe" concentration of these chemicals is "zero"—in other words, carcinogen-free water.

The Safe Drinking Water Act of 1974 empowered the Environmental Protection Agency to set mandatory standards for all chemicals contaminating drinking water and gave states the primary responsibility for enforcement. The act defines both federal and state obligations for safeguarding the quality of the nation's drinking water. This act covers all community water systems, even small ones that serve recreational areas, trailer parks, and commercial establishments. Under the act, the Environmental Protection Agency will set rules limiting both bacterial and chemical contaminants in the drinking water. Most systems will have to comply by 1976. In addition to providing federal funds to bolster state drinking water programs, the new act permits the EPA to prescribe specific water treatment procedures and to limit public exposure to certain contaminants even if they have not been conclusively proven to be harmful.

A potential weakness in the law, however, is that state governments are designated as the primary enforcers of the rules, and they may excuse existing systems from meeting certain of the new standards for up to nine years. The federal government has the authority to step in, but only after finding that the state "has, in a substantial number of instances, abused its discretion."

The technology is available for removing the carcinogens. All that is needed is further filtration of the water through activated charcoal filters. In fact, the city of Mount Clemens, Michigan, has been doing this since 1968. The original purpose was to remove bad-tasting chemicals from the water, but the carbon not only removes the bad-tasting chemicals, but the carcinogens as well, including the pesticides. The additional treatment of the water costs only about seven cents per month per resident—a small price to pay for the protection.

As early as 1972 a published study revealed that the Evansville, Indiana, municipal drinking water was loaded with organic chemicals. The water is taken from the Ohio River. Over forty different chemicals were detected by using several analysis techniques. Thirteen of the compounds were identified exactly as to chemical structure. The source of one of these chemicals was found to be an industrial plant 150 miles upstream. The thirteen chemicals positively identified were the following:

Bromodichloromethane
Toluene
Chlorodibromomethane
Tetrachloroethylene
Ethylbenzene
Xylene
Styrene
Bromoform
Bis (2-chloroethyl) ether
Bis (2-chloroisopropyl) ether
Hexachloroethane
Hexachlorobenzene
Chlorohydroxybenzophenone

Many of these chemicals have known toxic properties in higher concentrations than found in the drinking water. The most bothersome part of the problem is that the long-term effect of chronic exposure to these chemicals in the water is not known.

On November 8, 1974, the Environmental Protection Agency announced the results of its studies of the New Orleans drinking water. It found sixty-six different organic chemicals, at least eight of which are known or suspected toxic compounds, some of which cause cancer in animals. The eight most dangerous of these chemicals are listed below:

Bromodichloromethane
Bromoform
Carbon tetrachloride
Bis (2-chloroethyl) ether
Chloroform
Bis (2-chloroisopropyl) ether
Dibromochloromethane
1,2-dichloroethane

Among the other chemicals found in the drinking water were the insecticides dieldrin and eldrin, carbon disulfide, ethanol, hexachloroethane, methanol, and triphenyl phosphate. Of the foregoing chemicals, five are known to be carcinogenic in laboratory animals: carbon tetrachloride, chloroform, bis (2-chloroethyl) ether, dieldrin, and eldrin.

Follow-up studies of the New Orleans water contamination problem have shown that residents of the city have measurable levels of suspected cancer-causing chemicals in their blood. Biologists at the University of New Orleans studied both drinking water and blood samples of residents and found two chemicals that were present in both. These were carbon tetrachloride, a known carcinogen in animals, and tetrachloroethylene, a suspected carcinogen. The carbon tetrachloride was found at much higher concentrations in the blood than in the water, suggesting either that the chemical is accumulating in the body, probably in fat, or else that there is a source other than the drinking water, most likely the food supply. (This is likely, because many food manufacturing processes use organic solvents during processing. As mentioned earlier, for example, decaffeinated coffee is treated with trichloroethylene, and small amounts of the chemical are known to remain in the finished product.)

The potential hazard posed by the presence of chemical carcinogens in the drinking water was illustrated in a study performed by the Environmental Defense Fund, a Washington-based public interest group. The study showed that the incidence of cancer of the stomach, intestines, and urinary system was well above the national average in New Orleans. These are the organs most exposed to drinking water. Although no cause-and-effect relationship has been proven, suspicion among scientists runs high.

Out of 2,600 samples of drinking water from across the nation, EPA tests have revealed that 996, more than one-third, had unsafe levels of chemical or bacterial contamination. Other known or suspected cancer-causing agents found in the water include asbestos, arsenic, cadmium, benzene, cyanide, lead, and mercury.

This all adds up to the fact that millions of Americans may be drinking unsafe water, and the problem is getting worse with time.

An ad hoc study group for the Hazardous Materials Advisory Committee of the Science Advisory Board, a public advisory group providing scientific information to the administrator and other officials of the Environmental Protection Agency, has studied the problem of trace amounts of carcinogens in drinking water and has issued a report of its findings. This study group was composed of eminent scientists from the nation's leading universities.

In the report, issued April 30, 1975, the study group stated that any assessment of possible human health risk associated with consumption of drinking water contaminated with low concentrations of organic chemicals depends on at least three factors: (1) the adequacy of analytic methods for identifying and measuring the contaminants and the scope of their application, (2) the existence and adequacy of toxicological data on the contaminants, and (3) the extent to which appropriate epidemiologic studies have been conducted to test a hypothesis of association derived from the water quality data and the toxicological data. The study group addressed itself to these issues, with carcinogenesis as the toxic effect of primary concern. The group recognized that a complete assessment of the possible risk should include those risks associated with exposure to other contaminants such as pesticides, asbestos, and inorganic chemicals, all of which were explicitly excluded from the charge of the study group.

With respect to assessment of health risk associated with exposure to the specific contaminants with which it was dealing, the study group concluded that some human health risk does exist. The conclusion was based on evidence that some of the compounds, particularly chloroform, are widespread contaminants of drinking water supplies in the United States, and that studies in laboratory animals indicate that chloroform produces liver tumors. The study group emphasized that experimental carcinogenesis data for chloroform are extremely limited, although support for its tumorigenicity is reinforced by more extensive studies demonstrating carcinogenic action of the related compound, carbon tetrachloride. These two compounds probably act by a similar mechanism to produce liver tumors. Carbon tetrachloride, although occasionally identified as a contaminant of drinking water, occurs generally at much lower concentrations and is much less widespread as a contaminant than chloroform and related trihalogenated compounds. Benzene has not been clearly established to be carcinogenic in experimental animals, although epidemiologic and clinical studies strongly suggest its possible carcinogenicity. Certain haloethers, chlorolefins, and polynuclear hydrocarbons have been demonstrated to be carcinogenic in laboratory animals, and have been identified in drinking water. To the very limited extent that they have been measured, the data available to the study group indicate that the potential human dosage of these compounds from ingestion of drinking water will generally be considerably less in absolute quantities as well as relative to experimentally carcinogenic doses in laboratory animals than for chloroform. However, the study group noted the existence of local situations in which this generalization would not apply.

The study group felt that for all the chemicals reviewed, the carcinogenicity data and experimental designs were generally either inappropriate or below the standard of current toxicologic practice and protocols for carcinogenicity testing. Additional well-designed experiments to determine the carcinogenicity of lifetime exposures to these chemicals were sorely needed.

7
Home, Sweet Home

Oh, beautiful, for spacious skies
For amber waves of grain
For purple mountains' majesty
Above the fruited plain
America, America!
God shed His grace on thee . . .

—America the Beautiful
Katharine Lee Bates

Beautiful words to a beautiful song! One cannot help but think of them while driving on westbound I-94 through the summer wheat fields of North Dakota, into the Big Sky country of Montana, where the sky seems bigger and bluer than anywhere else on the continent. In western Montana the mountains come into view. I-94 becomes I-90 and passes through several towns nestled in valleys. One cannot help thinking that this must be an ideal, healthy place to live. It has beautiful, clear skies, clean air, pure water, and nice people.

Continuing on I-90 westbound, the road starts a steep

upgrade. At the top a sign states that we are entering Silver Bow County. A short distance west another sign tells us that we have just crossed the Continental Divide. After a steep downgrade a town comes into view. "What a swell place to live!" must have crossed the minds of many travelers as they started the descent into the city of Butte, Montana.

Such thoughts quickly go up in smoke, however, as the traveler descends the final curve through the mountain and sees the entire city for the first time. It is engulfed in an ugly brown cloud, and just to the right of the city, half a mountain has been mined.

The acrid smell of the brown cloud becomes evident several miles from the city. The traveler must wonder how the people of Butte can stand living in this environment year after year. But mining is the entire economy of Butte, and the people have to live with it or face economic collapse.

In the 1880s Butte became known as "the richest hill on earth." Placer gold was discovered in 1864, and silver was first extracted in 1875. Silver production declined markedly after the price dropped in 1893. Copper production began in Butte in 1882 and by 1900 represented 50 percent of the nation's output. Other minerals from the mines of Butte include zinc, lead, and manganese.

In an effort to relieve the chronic instability in the Butte economy, the Anaconda Copper Mining Company in 1952 adopted a twenty-year plan called the Greater Butte Project, followed in 1955 by the beginning of open-pit operations in the Berkeley mine, which is what we saw to the right of the city when entering.

What about the health of the people of Butte? Does living in this brown cloud affect their longevity? Is morbidity associated with it, or is it just a harmless eyesore?

Studies of the causes of death among Butte residents have revealed that both men and women have a high incidence of lung cancer. Men also die of stomach cancer more frequently than expected.

One source of the heavy air pollution in Butte is the sanding material used on city streets during the winter months to aid traction for automobiles. This material is a soft, decomposed quartz that is ground by automobile traffic to a dust that blankets the entire city during dry periods. This quartz has the same composition as the waste rock from the mines. It contains a number of silicates similar in chemical structure to asbestos. The types of lung cancer found in the men and women of Butte closely match those found among asbestos workers. For this reason, scientists suspect that the dust may be the carcinogen responsible for the Butte lung cancer.

About twenty-five miles northwest of Butte is the city of Anaconda, Montana. With a population of about 10,000, it is the seat of Deer Lodge County. In Anaconda is a smelter with a 585-foot smokestack that dominates the landscape. This smelter creates significant air pollution in the city. Atmospheric surveys have revealed a marked increase in arsenic and a moderate increase in lead levels as compared to other Montana cities and other major cities of the United States. In addition, industrial hygiene surveys have found high concentrations of sulfur dioxide, oxides of nitrogen, copper, zinc, manganese, arsenic, lead, and cadmium in working areas of the smelter.

Anaconda men and women also appear to have a high incidence of lung cancer, but it is of a different type than that seen among the people of Butte. Scientists attribute the Anaconda lung cancer to chronic exposure to airborne arsenic.

Variations in the geographical distribution of different types of cancer provide leads to the causes of the disease. A study by Dr. Thomas Mason and his colleagues at the Epidemiology Branch of the National Cancer Institute resulted in a 1975 publication entitled *Atlas of Cancer Mortality for U.S. Counties: 1950–1969* (DHEW Publication No. 75-780). This atlas revealed striking findings regarding the incidence of cancer in various part of the United States. Silver Bow and Deer Lodge Counties in Montana are just two of many examples.

Of the twenty-one counties in New Jersey, eighteen have male bladder cancer rates that are among the highest in the country. In fact, Salem County, New Jersey, has the highest rate (16.1 per 100,000 population) of all American counties with a white population of at least 100,000. In this county approximately one-fourth of the work force is employed in chemical and allied industries, suggesting that the bladder cancer is occupationally related. However, cancer of the colon and rectum in this area, and in the entire northeast section of the United States, occurs at a high rate in both males and females, suggesting causative or contributory factors common to both sexes, such as diet.

An area that seems an unlikely high-cancer region is Saint Louis County, Minnesota. This area, however, has high rates for both sexes of cancer of the stomach, pancreas, kidneys, and thyroid, plus multiple myeloma and leukemia. In males, rates are high for cancer of the nasopharnyx, esophagus, and rectum and for Hodgkin's disease; in females, rates are high for cancer of the liver, brain, nervous system, and ovary and for lymphosarcoma and reticulosarcoma. The seat of Saint Louis County is Duluth, Minnesota, the western terminal of the Saint Lawrence Seaway. Harbor facilities include coal docks, grain elevators, and iron ore docks that receive taconite. Major industries include a steel mill and a blast furnace, which probably contribute to the high cancer rate. Furthermore, asbestos from Lake Superior is known to contaminate the drinking water of Duluth residents, a fact that also may contribute to the high cancer rate.

The National Cancer Institute study revealed other striking differences in the geographical patterns of cancer mortality. The Northeast (New Jersey, southern New York, Connecticut, Rhode Island, and Massachusetts) and urban areas along the Great Lakes (Buffalo, Cleveland, Detroit, Chicago, and Milwaukee) had high rates of cancer of the large intestine and rectum in both sexes; of mouth, throat, esophagus, larynx, and bladder in males; and of the breast in females. These same malignancies occurred with low frequency in the southern and central parts of the United States.

The southern United States and Appalachia had high rates of skin cancer in both sexes, while females had high rates of cancer of the lip, mouth, throat, esophagus, cervix, eyes, and bones. These cancers had a low incidence in the Northeast.

The north central states (the Dakotas, Minnesota, Wisconsin, and Upper Michigan) had high death rates from cancer of the stomach and kidney as well as for multiple myeloma and leukemia in both sexes. Prostrate cancer was high in males, while lymphosarcoma and reticulosarcoma were high in females.

The rural North had high rates of testicular cancer and lymphosarcoma and reticulosarcoma in males, while ovarian and bladder cancer were high in females. These same tumors had a low incidence in the South.

There were no clearly discernible geographical patterns for cancer of the brain and nervous system, pancreas, salivary glands, nose and sinuses, and connective tissue.

These patterns in the National Cancer Institute cancer mortality study occurred through 1969. Excluding skin tumors, the majority of these cancers are thought to have been caused by exposure to chemical carcinogens, and the exposure responsible for these malignancies occurred years before diagnosis. Since thousands of untested new chemicals have been introduced into various areas of our country in the past twenty years, these geographical patterns of cancer mortality will undoubtedly change somewhat.

It is now possible to predict intelligently some of these changes. All areas of the country will probably have overall increases in cancer due to exposure to chemical carcinogens in consumer products. Cancer rates in the industrial Northeast and Great Lakes urban centers will continue to be high. The Great Lakes states will probably experience increases due to local consumption of fish and other foods contaminated with polychlorinated biphenyls and insecticides. Michigan in particular may have increased rates of liver and other cancers due to the widespread contamination of livestock with polybrominated biphenyls and contaminants. Populations along the western shore of Lake Superior may have increased rates of gastrointestinal and other cancers due to the contamination of drinking water and air with asbestos. The low cancer rates in Colorado, Wyoming, and most of Montana will very likely yield to increases in lung cancer following development of coal mining and petroleum refining.

In general, any area with heavy industry, chemicals, certain mining oprations, petroleum refining, or agriculture using large quantities of insecticides can expect increases in cancer, and no area is likely to escape some increase in cancer due to exposure of populations to carcinogens in consumer products.

8
Naturally
Occuring
Carcinogens

Not all chemical carcinogens are man-made. Nature has provided a number of naturally occurring carcinogens that have been around for a long time. Many of these compounds are produced by various members of the plant kingdom while others are products of naturally occurring phenomena.

Fungi, or molds, produce a number of astonishingly potent metabolic products. Some of these products, including penicillin and chloromycetin, are beneficial to man. However, scientists are becoming increasingly aware of the existence of harmful substances called mycotoxins, also produced by molds. Certain molds growing on foods can produce mycotoxins with disastrous effects. The dangers of some mycotoxins have been known for a long time because they act rapidly, making clear the association between ingestion of contaminated food and the onset of symptoms. A good example is the ergot fungus that grows on rye. Repeated consumption of contaminated rye causes an affliction known as Saint Anthony's fire. The disease is characterized by behavioral changes and sometimes by gangrene of the fingers and toes due to prolonged contraction of smooth muscle fibers in the walls of blood vessels. There is a rapid onset of symptoms.

On the other hand, scientists now realize that some mycotoxins may produce cancer, but as with other carcinogens, the process may take years to manifest itself. One group of mycotoxins, the aflatoxins, are known to produce liver cancer in animals. Some data suggest that aflatoxins also produce liver cancer in humans.

The aflatoxins were discovered in the early 1960s after 100,000 turkeys died after eating peanut meal. Analysis of the meal revealed contamination with the mold *Aspergillus flavus*. Extracts of the mold, when fed to more turkeys, had the same toxic effect. It was later found that the substance, an aflatoxin, produced liver cancer in rats.

Since that time aflatoxins have been found in a variety of other human and animal foods, including rice, wheat, pepper, and wine. However, peanuts are the most likely source of aflatoxins in the human diet. In areas where peanuts are harvested when they have a high moisture content and when no precautions such as rapid drying are taken against mold formation, as much as 75 percent of the crop may contain the *Aspergillus* mold. Large producers of peanuts in the United States employ rigid measures to prevent contamination of their products by aflatoxins. However, the instrumentation necessary to check samples is costly, and many small companies do not check their products routinely. Needless to say, the consumer is much safer if he limits his consumption of peanut products to those manufactured by the largest companies.

The two major types of aflatoxins are named aflatoxin B (blue) and aflatoxin G (green) after the color of their fluorescence under ultraviolet light. Aflatoxin B^1 is the compound of greatest importance because it occurs commonly and has the highest toxicity. In fact, aflatoxin B^1 is the most potent carcinogen yet discovered. A dose as low as 0.0004 gram can cause liver cancer in rats.

The carcinogenic effect of aflatoxins was first described in rats, but further studies have produced aflatoxin-induced tumors in ducks, trout, guinea pigs, and rhesus monkeys.

Other products of molds have been shown to produce

cancer. Mycotoxins from a type of penicillin that contaminates yellowed rice has been shown to produce liver cancer in mice. Undoubtedly, future research will demonstrate other carcinogens from other molds.

In addition to the mycotoxins, many other natural carcinogens are produced by plants. Dr. Erich Hecker of the West German government's cancer research center has recently identified five house and garden plants that produce cancer-causing chemicals. These chemicals are called co-carcinogens and cause the second phase of a two-stage process leading to the development of cancer. The first step occurs when one is exposed to a chemical carcinogen such as vinyl chloride. The person will not get cancer at that time, but rather much later, after the latent period has passed. Furthermore, if the person were exposed to less than a critical dose, he would not develop the cancer at all. However, if the person comes in contact with a co-carcinogen any time after being exposed to the carcinogen (in this case, the vinyl chloride), he will develop the cancer much faster. Even if he had been exposed to a subcritical dose of the carcinogen, and then to the co-carcinogen, he would still get the cancer.

Testing for the activity of co-carcinogens is interesting. A typical procedure consists of a one-time painting of a carcinogen (let's use coal tar) on the skin of a group of mice. The dose is known to be too small to cause cancer. Another group of mice gets the same treatment once a week for thirteen weeks. These mice will not get cancer either because the dose is too small. But if a third group of mice gets painted with the carcinogen only once, and then has twelve weekly applications of the co-carcinogen, the mice will develop cancer. A fourth group of mice, painted only with the co-carcinogen, will not get cancer. The two chemicals must interact in some way for the malignancy to develop.

Co-carcinogens are of great importance to man. For example, a person who has smoked for twenty years, exposing himself to tobacco smoke carcinogens, decides to stop. But he has already subjected himself to the first stage. If he later comes in contact with a co-carcinogen, he may increase his chances of getting the disease.

Evidence of the existence of naturally occurring co-carcinogens is growing. Dr. Benjamin Van Duuren of New York University identified a co-carcinogen in croton oil several years ago. Now Dr. Hecker warns of the presence of other co-carcinogens in five plants, several of which are popular garden species in the United States. These plants are commonly known as (1) the crown of thorns or "thorns of Christ," (2) the pencil tree, (3) the caper spurge, (4) the candelabra cactus, and (5) the coral plant.

At present fifteen plants are known to produce co-carcinogens. Six of these grow in the United States. (The sixth is the machineel.)

The first five plants cited are all grown commercially and shipped around the country. The crown of thorns (Euphorbia millii) is a thorny bush with green leaves and small red flowers. The pencil tree (Euphorbia tirucalli) is a green plant that grows to eight feet in height and has pencillike branches. It is also known as the milk bush, Indian tree, pencil cactus, malabar tree, monkey fiddle, and spurge. The caper spurge (Euphorbia lathyris) is a green plant that grows to six feet in height and has yellow flowers. It is also known as the mole plant, garden spurge, myrtle spurge, mole weed, gopher plant, and springwort. The candelabra cactus (Euphorbia lactea) is a green thorny plant. The coral plant (Jatropha multifida) is a small tree with pink flowers. It is also known as the physic nut.

Certain foods themselves produce carcinogens. The cycad nut, used to produce flour by the peoples of Guam and Japan, has been found to contain a very potent carcinogen. The chemical, called cycasin, is so potent that just one dose can produce tumors in experimental animals. Fortunately, this chemical is washed out of the flour during its preparation of human consumption.

Another plant containing a carcinogenic substance is the braken fern. It has been suggested that the use of braken for human consumption in Japan may be responsible for the high incidence of stomach cancer in that country. The young braken fronds generally used for food usually are processed by various forms of cooking, involving immersion in boiling water. Studies with rats revealed that cooking decreases the carcinogenic properties of brakens but does not abolish them entirely. Other studies have shown that the carcinogenic component is passed into the milk of cows fed this fern. Scientists suspect that braken ferns may also contain a mutagenic substance.

Another nut, the betel nut, also is suspected of containing a carcinogen. In the Orient this nut is chewed by natives in certain localities. These people have a high incidence of cancer of the mouth. Research has demonstrated the presence of several suspected carcinogens in the nuts.

On the Caribbean island of Curacao, esophageal cancer accounts for 18 percent of all cancers, and stomach cancer accounts for 16 percent. It has been noted that a high proportion of the people with esophageal cancer had a history of frequent intake of local herbal medicines and teas. On the nearby island of Aruba, the use of local medicinal plants is much less, and the incidence of esophageal cancer is quite small. Scientists are checking the local herbal medicines of Curacao and so far have found some evidence of the presence of carcinogens.

Another naturally occurring carcinogen is found in wood smoke. It is called benz (a) pyrene, and we eat it regularly in a number of foods. A survey of benz (a) pyrene in the American diet has revealed 4.5 parts per billion in barbecued pork, 3.2 ppb in cured ham, and 6.9 ppb in smoked fish. Charcoal-broiled meats were by far the most highly contaminated, with 10.5 ppb in barbecued ribs and 50 ppb in some T-bone steaks. It was found that the proximity of the meat to the charcoal was an important factor—the closer the meat the higher the level of benz (a) pyrene.

Benz (a) pyrene causes cancer in a number of animals. It is one of the most ubiquitous carcinogens in our environment and could conceivably be responsible for a significant proportion of human cancers, although the human effect has yet to be determined, and the effects of inhalation exposure in animals has yet to be studied.

Benz (a) pyrene also occurs naturally in crude oil, and has been identified in a number of petroleum products, including commercial gasoline.

9
Polychlorinated Biphenyls

Imagine yourself on the banks of the Platt River outside Traverse City, Michigan. It is springtime. The trout and salmon are coming up the river from Lake Michigan to spawn. The leaves are just out on the trees, the sun is shining, and the river is crystal clear. You can see all the salmon swimming in the river! Everything is peaceful and tranquil. It is is good to get away from the city and be here where the air is clean and smells good.

You cast your line in the river. A strike! A big one! You haul him in—a big coho salmon. You can't wait to take him home, cook him, and sit down to a delicious fish dinner, right? Wrong! If you're smart, you won't eat that fish. He's loaded with polychlorinated biphenyls—up to 165 parts per million, to be more specific. Polychlorinated biphenyls are known to cause cancers in rats. The recommended upper limit for safe eating established by the FDA in 1973 is only 5 ppm, and recent studies suggest that PCBs may be hazardous at the stipulated level or lower.

How did that happen, you ask? And how did coho salmon

get into Lake Michigan in the first place? It is all part of the story of the decline of Lake Michigan. The name Michigan was derived from the Algonquin Indian words *michi,* meaning great, and *gami,* meaning water. The lake was indeed once a great water— pure and clean, teeming with edible gamefish. Then the white man came, building steel mills, factories, and chemical plants, pouring pollutants into the crystal clear waters. Then came the St. Lawrence Seaway, mixing the ecology of the saltwater ocean with the freshwater lake. As mentioned, the lamprey eel came in through the seaway, destroying millions more gamefish. Then came the alewives—thin, inedible fish which essentially replaced the perch.

The Michigan Department of Natural Resources was very concerned about the disaster that struck Lake Michigan. The DNR valiantly tried to come up with a partial solution to the problem. The commercial fishing industry had been virtually wiped out, so the department decided to import a new type of fish that would restore the industry and at the same time revive Michigan's once-famous game fishing. The answer seemed to be the coho salmon, imported from the northwestern United States. The coho grows to a large size fairly rapidly and had the added advantage that each one would eat a remarkable number of the undesirable alewives.

However, the Department of Natural Resources staff did not consider the presence of the polychlorinated biphenyls that had been dumped into the lake over the past forty years.

Polychlorinated biphenyls, or PCBs, have become widespread environmental contaminants. They belong to a class of chemicals that have a number of toxic properties. For the benefit of readers with some background in chemistry, the structures of PCBs and their relatives are diagrammed in Figure 2. Two hundred and ten chlorine-substituted biphenyls can be created by the placement of chlorine atoms at the various corners of the carbon rings. Several of the chemical relatives of PCBs illustrated may be present as contaminants in PCB products.

Perhaps the most distressing thing about polychlorinated biphenyls is that they are relatively nonbiodegradable. They are slowly accumulating in rivers and seas. They are used in plastics,

Figure 2
Some Polychlorinated Biphenyls and Related Chemicals

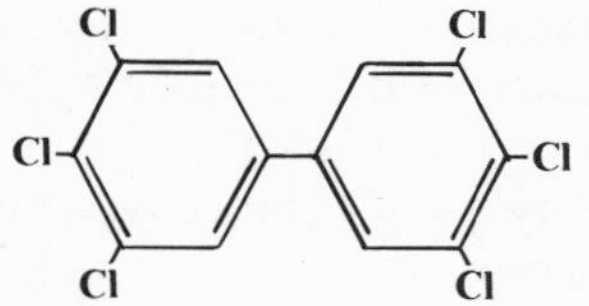

Polychlorinated Biphenyls
(PCB)

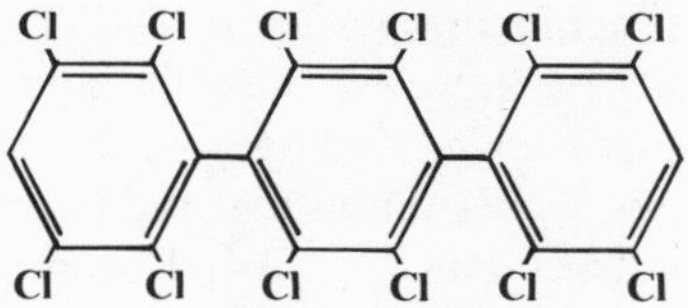

Polychlorinated Terphenyl

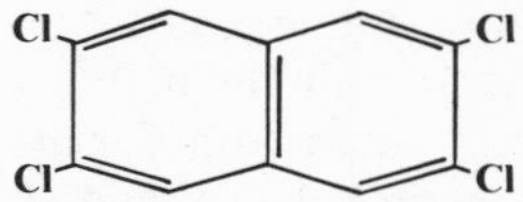

Polychlorinated Naphthalene

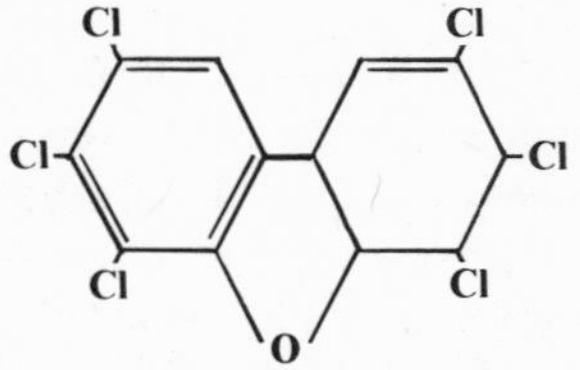

Polychlorinated Dibenzofuran

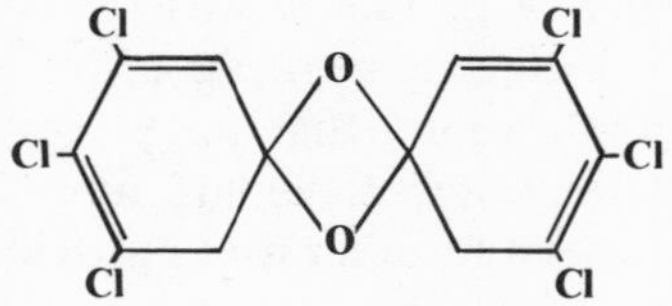

Polychlorinated Dibenzodioxin

paints, sealants, adhesives, and printing inks, escaping into the environment from sewage and industrial effluent. The predominant uses of PCBs prior to 1971, in order of importance, were for capacitors, plasticizer applications including use in carbonless duplicating paper, transformer liquids, hydraulic fluids, lubricants, and heat-transfer liquids.

PCBs are found in the fat stores of numerous animals, including man. The long-term chronic toxicity of PCBs in man is not fully understood. However, the marked accumulation of any compound such as this must be considered cause for concern.

Polychlorinated biphenyls were introduced into industry in 1929. They were not identified as widespread environmental contaminants until 1966 and they did not generate any great concern until several episodes attracted attention to their wide distribution and potential hazard to health. PCBs resemble the organochlorine pesticides (DDT, for example) in their ability to persist in the environment, and they are easily confused with these pesticides during analysis by gas chromatography.

PCBs are manufactured by the chlorination of biphenyl with anhydrous chlorine using iron filings as a catalyst. The sole producer in the United States and the world's leading supplier is the Monsanto Corporation, which sells the product under the trade name Aroclors. The cumulative production of PCBs by 1972 in the United States alone was estimated at 500,000 tons. PCBs are also manufactured in Great Britain, France, Germany, the USSR, Japan, Italy, Spain, and Czechoslovakia.

PCB pollution is a global problem. It has been estimated that in 1972 the *cumulative* input of PCBs into the oceans around North America alone from the combination of local discharge and aerial fallout was 15,000 tons.

Several years ago, Monsanto began refusing to sell PCBs for applications that might cause widespread environmental contamination. Sales are now limited to use in electronic components and other areas providing minimal possibility of introduction into the environment. These restrictions should eventually reduce the accumulation of these compounds in the environment.

However, PCBs persist in human foodstuffs. The average daily intake of a person in the United States is estimated at 0.1 microgram per kilogram per day. The main source is fish.

PCBs have been found to contaminate foods in ways other than through the food chain. They were used as sealants for silos, thus contaminating silage. Cows fed the silage had PCBs in their milk. PCBs also were used in food processing plants, thus further contaminating food sources.

Food packaging materials made from recycled paper containing carbonless copying paper and printing inks are further sources of food contamination. One sample of ground cashew nuts was tested and found to contain 10 ppm PCBs. This sample had been shipped in a lacquered cardboard drum, which on analysis proved to contain 200 ppm of the same PCB.

In 1968 contamination of cooking oil in Japan resulted in

PCB poisoning of over a thousand people. The predominant symptom was severe, persistent skin lesions. The same accidental contamination also resulted in adulterated chicken feed, causing the death of a large number of chickens. A second episode of contamination of chicken feed occurred in the United States in 1971.

In 1969 large-scale mortality of fish-eating birds in Great Britain led to the discovery of significant levels of PCBs in fish used for human consumption. Numerous studies of PCB distribution in the environment soon followed.

It was found that PCBs enter the food chain from lakes and rivers through their ingestion by aquatic animals and the subsequent ingestion of aquatic animals by birds. The more highly chlorinated PCBs have an extremely low solubility in water and are found mostly in the sediment at the bottom of the sea.

PCBs have been found in concentrations of up to 120 ppm in shrimp and 1.5 ppm in crabs from the Escambia Bay area of Florida. PCBs were found mainly in the sediment in the bay. The source apparently was a chemical plant somewhat upstream. It was further demonstrated that the shrimp and crabs could concentrate the PCBs until the levels in their tissues exceeded the levels of contamination on the sea bottom. Contamination of fish from the area appeared to be somewhat lower, ranging around 1 ppm.

In an experiment, fish kept in water contaminated with known concentrations of PCBs were found to accumulate levels of PCB much higher than that of the water. For example, a concentration of 5 parts per *billion* in the water resulted in levels of over 100 parts per *million* in fish. This concentration was fatal to over 50 percent of the subjects. If the surviving fish were then transferred to nonpolluted water, the PCB levels in their tissues fell by about 73 percent after three months.

PCB levels also have been measured in animals and birds in Great Britain. Concentrations in livers of fish-eating birds reached 900 ppm. Eighty ppm were found in herons' eggs. These eggs also contained insecticides (26.5 ppm DDE and 6.5 ppm dieldrin). PCBs are moderately toxic to fish, and to some aquatic invertebrates at levels as low as 1 part per *billion!*

Other animals have been found to accumulate polychlorinated biphenyls. An extreme example is the grey seal, whose body fat commonly contains from 10–50 ppm PCB but may contain as much as 1,800 ppm. Of importance to man is the finding of PCBs in commercial food supplies. Commercial fish oils contain up to 3 ppm and levels of less that 1 ppm have been found in margarines manufactured from vegetable and marine oils.

Most human exposure to PCBs appears to be by ingestion of contaminated fish. Occasional contamination of other foods such as milk and poultry have led to significantly higher intakes for short periods. Mean levels of PCBs in human fat average about 1 ppm in the United States and 6 ppm in Germany. However, human exposure and fat concentrations of PCBs vary considerably. One investigator reported discovery of up to 200 ppm PCBs in house dust in Michigan, and fat levels of three Michigan residents taken at autopsy measured 200 ppm, 240 ppm, and 600 ppm respectively! Human milk has been found to contain up to 3.5 ppm PCBs.

Toxicological studies of polychlorinated biphenyls are complicated because of the large number of different chlorinated biphenyls present in most mixtures. The term *polychlorinated biphenyls* refers to a mixture of many different PCB compounds. As mentioned earlier, 210 different compounds are possible. Furthermore, highly toxic impurities have been found in some batches of PCBs.

Several investigators have found marked differences in toxicity between three commercial preparations of PCBs with the same degree of chlorination. The more toxic batches were found to contain impurities, including tetra- and pentachlorodibenzofurans and hexa- and heptachloronaphthalenes. The pentachlorodibenzofurans were present in concentrations as high as 20 ppm.

The toxic effects of PCBs vary widely throughout the animal kingdom. Levels as low as 1 ppb are toxic to some fish and the pink shrimp. Chickens fed 100–150 ppm in the diet for up to five weeks gained less weight than expected, exhibited swelling, breathlessness, internal hemorrhages, depression of secondary sex characteristics, and increased liver weights. At levels of 50 ppm, these changes were less marked, and at 10 ppm no signs or symptoms were present. However, in another study, behavioral changes were seen in robins receiving as little as 5 micrograms daily in the diet.

In another study, rats fed PCBs showed that the less chlorinated components were metabolized more than the more highly chlorinated components.

Pregnant rabbits fed 10 milligrams PCB per kilogram of weight per day had normal offspring. However, increasing the dose to 12.5 milligrams per kilogram per day throughout the pregnancy led to an increase in abortions and stillbirths. Rats appeared to be less sensitive in a study conducted by Monsanto. Concentrations of Aroclors had no effect at 1 and 10 parts per million, but at 100 ppm, second generation animals had increased stillbirth rates. Reduced mating has also been reported in rats fed PCBs. In other studies embryotoxicity has been reported in both rabbits and birds.

A study of monkeys showed liver changes characteristic of an increase in enzymatic activity and degeneration of livers after consumption of PCBs. In another study, rabbits treated with PCBs were found to have liver hypertrophy, damage to the kidney tubules, decreased white blood counts, and atrophy of the thymus gland. In this study PCBs were applied to the skin five times a week for thirty-eight days. The skin itself developed lesions characterized by hyperplasia and hyperkeratosis.

Very little work on metabolism of PCBs has been performed. There is some evidence that lower PCBs (four or fewer chlorine atoms per molecule) are metabolized fairly rapidly. Higher PCBs are more refractory, although some PCBs with five or six chlorine atoms per molecule appear to be metabolized by birds and mammals. PCBs can cause liver changes at dietary levels as low as 0.5 ppm, suggesting that even low residues in the environment could pose a threat to health.

In long-term toxicity experiments with PCBs, several harmful effects on the liver have been observed. Effects on sex hormones have been reported in rats and birds. Some of these effects increased with increasing chlorine content of the PCBs, while others decreased. Experts suggest that some of the observed toxic effects are due to the PCBs or their metabolites while others are due to contaminants.

An immunosuppressive effect from PCBs is suggested by a number of observations. Lymphopenia has been reported in rabbits, and decreases in numbers of antibody-forming cells have been reported in guinea pigs treated with PCBs.

Mutagenic effects of PCBs also are of concern. Second-generation doves fed PCBs (Aroclors 1254) exhibited a high frequency of chromosomal aberrations. However, human studies so far have been negative.

A study of the carcinogenicity of PCBs was recently completed by Dr. Renate Kimbrough, a pathologist and toxicologist at the Center for Disease Control in Atlanta. In her study she fed 100 ppm of a commercial preparation of PCBs (Aroclors 1260) to Sherman rats for twenty-one months. The rats were then killed and autopsied. Table 1 shows the results.

Table 1
Effects of PCBs on Rats

Disease	Incidence in Controls (N=173)	Incidence in Experimental Subjects (N=184)
Hepatocellular carcinoma (liver cancer)	1	26
Neoplastic nodules (early liver cancer)	0	144
Areas of atypical cells (precancerous)	28	182

Kimbrough's study shows that PCBs are definitely carcinogenic in rats. In other long-term studies, it was found that PCBs accumulate in tissues, and even after feeding for 240 days the levels did not reach a plateau. The half-life was found to be more than thirty days.

Recent studies by Dr. James R. Allen from the University of Wisconsin's Primate Research Center revealed that rhesus monkeys, only a few months after starting diets containing as little as 2.5 parts per million polychlorinated biphenyls, suffered loss of hair, skin lesions, general metabolic disturbances, menstrual irregularities, and gastrointestinal problems. Low levels of PCBs in the diet also apparently caused abortions and sickly offspring. These studies raise the possibility that if man were exposed to similar levels for the same time period, he also might become extremely ill.

In 1968 a group of people was accidentally poisoned in Japan. They ate rice cooked in oil contaminated with about 2,000 ppm PCBs. Although the oil itself was highly contaminated, the total dose of each person was low because the oil in the rice constituted only a small fraction of their total diet. The PCBs appeared to have caused severe symptoms at levels lower than the amounts needed to produce symptoms in experimental animals, indicating either that humans are more sensitive to the chemicals or that it was actually contaminants (dibenzofurans) in the PCBs that caused many of the symptoms. Many experts favor the latter theory.

This outbreak of PCB poisoning became known as the "Yusho" incident. Of the 1,000 persons poisoned with PCBs, 189 were subjected to intense clinical study. Chloracne (skin rash), hypersecretion of the Meibomian glands, hyperpigmentation of the skin, and transient reduction of growth in male children were noted. Some patients made little progress even after three years had passed. Symptoms were slow to appear, taking from five to six months to manifest themselves following ingestion of the chemicals. Various other symptoms were noted, including headache, vomiting, diarrhea, numbness, weakness, swelling of limbs, eye discharge, and swelling of the eyelids. Of thirteen pregnant women, two gave birth to stillborn children. Liveborn infants had dark brown skin pigmentation, dark nails and gums, and increased eye discharge. A study of four of the infants born to mothers with PCB poisoning revealed that the frontal and occipital fontanelles were abnormally large, and the sagittal suture was abnormally wide. Their faces were swollen, and three had exophthalmia (protruding eyes).

PCBs appear to alter fat metabolism in humans. Many of the Yusho cases had elevated serum triglycerides, and increased 17-ketosteroid excretion was noted.

In the 1940s in the United States an outbreak of a new disease in cattle was reported. The disease was characterized by emaciation, liver degeneration, kidney damage, and dry, wrinkled, mange-like thickening of the skin (hyperkeratosis). Wartlike swellings occurred on the muzzle, gums, tongue, and esophagus, and the animals had stomach ulcers and intermittent diarrhea. They also displayed reduced milk production and spontaneous abortion. The malady was observed in at least thirty-five states, chiefly in the South and Midwest. For lack of a better name, the malady was termed "X-disease."

In 1949 a research program was instituted to study the cause and symptoms of X-disease. By 1950 scientists had proved that the malady could be produced by a toxic substance in feed pellets. Of 150 calves fed the pellets, 130 developed the skin manifestations of X-disease, and 47 died. It was observed that hyperkeratosis also developed in several calves that drank milk from affected cows.

In 1952 another scientist observed that calves licking a lubricant from the springs of trucks also developed the disease. He contacted the manufacturer and learned that the lubricant contained a chemical additive, chlorinated naphthalenes. The chlorinated naphthalenes are chemical relatives of PCBs and were subsequently proven to be the cause of X-disease.

It was then discovered that during their manufacture, feed pellets had been contaminated with grease from the bearings of machines. The grease contained chlorinated naphthalenes. Cows have also contracted the disease through exposure to chlorinated naphthalene–containing wood preservatives used on barns and from farm machines lubricated with oils containing the chemical.

An interesting environmental contamination problem that occurred recently in the Midwest involved the chemical trichlorophenol. A six-year-old girl had developed symptoms suggesting kidney disease, but the standard laboratory tests did not reveal the cause. She lived near a stable of horses and played in the riding arena. At the time of her illness, it happened that a number of sparrows and other birds that normally populated the barn rafters were found dead on the arena floor. Over the next several weeks, hundreds of birds, several dogs and cats, and numerous rodents died after being exposed to the arena. Of the 85 horses which were exercised for varying periods within the arena, 62 became ill and 48 died.

The Center for Disease Control in Atlanta was contacted. After thorough and exhaustive study of the problem, researchers found crystals of trichlorophenol in the soil of the area. Because they suspected that the toxic effects were actually due to a contaminant in the trichlorophenol, researchers performed further analysis and discovered 30 ppm of the extremely toxic chemical tetrachlorodibenzodioxin in the soil.

Further investigation revealed the source of both chemicals. A local company that recently had gone out of business had manufactured hexachlorophene. One of the waste products of the manufacturing process was an oil containing trichlorophenol and the contaminant tetrachlorodibenzodioxin. Before going out of business, the company had changed from one disposal company to another. The new disposal agent, not being aware of the chemical composition of the waste oil, used the oil to settle dust on roads and in riding arenas, thereby spreading tetrachlorodibenzodioxin all over the countryside!

The research team then went back to the buildings of the former chemical company and measured the concentrations of tetrachlorodibenzodioxin in the tank that held the waste oil. It measured over 300 ppm. The team then checked other riding arenas and roads in the area and found measurable levels.

The team postulated that the horses' symptoms were due to absorption of the chemicals through the hooves and to breathing TCDD–containing dust. Symptoms in horses from these arenas included weight loss, intestinal colic, oral ulcers, loss of hair, stiff hind legs, and staggering gait.

In addition to the girl, other humans in the area also complained of symptoms, including skin lesions, headaches, and joint pains.

The chemical tetrachlorodibenzodioxin is a well-known contaminant of the herbicide 2,4,5-T, which was used in Viet Nam. The contaminant—2,3,7,8-tetrachlorodibenzodioxin—is known to produce the following symptoms in animals: severe weight loss, hemorrhages, ulceration of the lining of the stomach, atrophy of the lymphatic system with depression of the immune response, liver damage, enzyme induction, chick edema disease, hyperkeratosis, birth defects, and fetal deaths.

The same contaminant is known to produce the following

symptoms in humans: skin lesions (chloracne), porphyria (a metabolic disease), liver damage, conjunctivitis, and birth defects.

The combination of dibenzofuran contaminants and PCBs is thought to have accounted for the symptoms in the people poisoned in the Yusho incident.

In the United States the Food and Drug Administration has set the acceptable daily limit of PCBs at 150–300 micrograms, and the maximum allowable concentration in fish at 5 ppm. Since 100 ppm polychlorinated biphenyls in the diet has recently been found to be carcinogenic in rodents, and other recent studies have shown deleterious effects in monkeys fed 2.5 ppm PCBs in the diet, it would seem prudent for the FDA to reconsider these guidelines.

A 1976 study of PCB levels in human breast milk revealed that concentrations of 5ppm and higher were common in the fat of milk from mothers living in industrial states. The effect of PCBs in human breast milk upon babies is unknown at this time. This latest finding has scientists concerned about the possible long-term effects of these concentrations of PCBs on the current generation of infants.

The true effects of PCBs and their contaminants on the human population, our rivers, lakes, and streams and on their plant and animal life will not be known for a number of years.

10
The Firemaster
Incident

For a three-year period, beginning in the summer of 1973, the population of Michigan was exposed to polybrominated biphenyls (PBBs) in milk and other dairy products, beef, chickens, eggs, pork, and other livestock products. The contamination occurred because of a series of errors resulting in the addition of the polybrominated biphenyls to livestock food.

The Michigan Chemical Corporation, a division of Northwest Industries, had been supplying the Michigan Farm Bureau Services with certain ingredients for livestock feed. One ingredient, magnesium oxide, was added to the feed to increase the fat content of milk from dairy cows. Michigan Chemical had a brand name, *Nutramaster,* for the chemical. In mid-1973, due to a shortage of packing bags, the color-coding system previously used to identify bags of different chemicals had been abandoned, and plain brown bags with the brand names of the products stenciled on them had been substituted for the printed bags. Another product, composed of polybrominated biphenyls and having the brand name *Firemaster*, had been sent to the Farm Bureau Services by mistake.

Employees at the Michigan Farm Bureau then mixed the polybrominated biphenyls with feed for dairy cows. The feed was distributed throughout Michigan and other areas. The machines used to mix the feed also were used to mix other types of livestock feed, thus resulting in contamination of other animals as well. This mistake resulted in the initial destruction of 6,000 cows, 900,000 chickens, 3,000,000 eggs, 2,300 pigs, and several thousand other animals and the chronic exposure of millions of people to low levels of polybrominated biphenyls in their diets. Destruction of thousands more animals followed as the true extent of the contamination became known.

In March 1975 depositions were taken from employees of the Michigan Farm Bureau Services to determine legal liability for the contamination of the millions of dollars' worth of livestock and the potential human injuries. The following is excerpted from these depositions:

Employee *A* was twenty-three years old when his deposition was taken on March 12, 1975. His last employer had been the Michigan Farm Bureau Services, but he had not worked for five months. His previous employment record was as unskilled labor. He had dropped out of school in the ninth grade.

He was given a fifteen-minute explanation of his job by the plant manager when he started working for the Farm Bureau in November 1969. His job was "catching bags" (receiving and unloading) in the warehouse. Part of his job was to unload bags of ingredients for farm feed from delivery trucks and to stack them in the warehouse. This included unloading bags of magnesium oxide from the Michigan Chemical Company.

Employee *A* admitted that he had not done well in school and that he could not read well enough to tell whether a bag had "Nutramaster" or "Firemaster" written on it.

Employee *B*, a resident of Kalamazoo, Michigan, started working at the Battle Creek feed-mixing plant in January 1971. His first job there was receiving the bulk ingredients for the feed. Bulk materials were received in one area of the plant and bagged materials in another. Sometimes, however, trucks carrying bulk materials would have bags of ingredients on them as well. When this happened, the bags would be loaded on skids and taken to the warehouse. Employee *B* worked in receiving for only a short time. Sometime before 1973 he was transferred to the mixing operation, where he mixed a number of ingredients to make the various feeds. About January 1974 he was transferred to a job driving a truck. He had never, prior to the Farm Bureau job, been engaged in the mixing of feed or feed products.

When Employee *B* started his new position as a mixer, the plant manager oriented him to the equipment he was to run. There were no written instructions or procedures for operating the mixer. The manager trained him for about a day and a half, and Employee *B* worked as a mixer for the entire year of 1973.

The mixer would put together a batch of feed by obtaining the proper ingredients, which were written on cards—a different card for each feed formula. Employee *B* occasionally asked *A* (who could not read very well) to go to the warehouse to obtain the required ingredients.

Bags of magnesium oxide had various brand names. Most bags from the several suppliers also had "magnesium oxide" or "mag ox" printed somewhere on the bag along with the brand name.

At one point *B* noticed that bags with "magnesium oxide" or "mag ox" printed on them were not available. He was told that bags labeled "Nutramaster" contained magnesium oxide and that he was to use those bags when the formula cards called for that particular chemical. *B* stated in his deposition that he would always ask one of his superiors about a product or ingredient he was not familiar with to make sure it was ok.

In June 1973 *B* was taking inventory in the warehouse. He noticed a stack of bags with the name "Firemaster" stenciled on them. He had never seen that brand before. He said he phoned the manager and asked him the difference between the new bags and Nutramaster. He said the manager told him that it was the same thing as Nutramaster and to put it with the Nutramaster and inventory it as magnesium oxide. The manager, according to *B*, did not check to determine whether there might have been a mix-up. He did not check the purchase order to see whether there had been a mistake.

As instructed, *B* picked up the Firemaster with the forklift and stacked it with the Nutramaster.

When he returned to his duties as a mixer, he began using the Firemaster as magnesium oxide. He knew the two labels were different, but as far as he was concerned, it was all right to use Firemaster because he had been told to do so.

In 1974, when the Firemaster incident became public, *B* had a new job driving a truck for the Michigan Farm Bureau Services. During the summer of 1974 he had a conversation with the manager. The term polybrominated biphenyls or PBB meant nothing to him, but when he heard the word Firemaster associated with the livestock contamination problem, he put two and two together. *B* asked the manager whether he remembered that he *(B)* had initially asked whether he should use the Firemaster. According to *B*, the manager said that he did not remember the telephone conversation or anything about the Firemaster. *B* remembered that the manager told him essentially, "Let's keep it in the company."

Employee *C* had worked at the Michigan Farm Bureau feed-mixing plant since 1969 when the facility opened. For the previous ten years he had worked for the Michigan Farm Bureau fertilizer plant in Kalamazoo as a mixer-operator. Altogether, he had worked for the Farm Bureau for sixteen years.

C described the bags of Nutramaster as plain brown bags with "Nutramaster" stenciled on them. When asked if the stenciling was clearly visible, he replied that it was clear on some of them but not on others. When asked how he knew that he was using a bag of Nutramaster if some of them had poor stenciling, he replied that the bags were all on the same skid. In other words, they were all *supposed* to be magnesium oxide. He assumed that the people responsible for stacking the bags put only magnesium oxide where magnesium oxide was supposed to be. He was told by the manager, he said, that "it was magnesium oxide, to use it as magnesium oxide, and that's all."

C remembered seeing bags of Firemaster on a skid in 1973. He denied ever using a bag of Firemaster when mixing feed himself, but he remembered seeing *B* using Firemaster in place of magnesium oxide while mixing. He questioned *B* about it, and *B* told him that he had gotten the OK to use it from the manager. At the same time, *C* stated that he himself had never personally received an OK to use Firemaster, so he refused to do so. He had noticed that the Firemaster material was "more powdery" than the material in the bags labeled Nutramaster. He stated that he personally was leery of the Firemaster.

After the contamination problem was discovered, the plant underwent a cleanup operation. According to *C*, employees were still mixing feed while the cleanup was in progress. The cleaning operation, he said, consisted of sweeping, blowing, and watering down the area with plain water. No soap or steam was used. Dust and debris collected during the cleanup were taken to the dump. *C* had participated in the cleaning of the mixer. The process was repeated several times. It consisted of chiseling the two-inch coating of residue from the sides of the mixer and the ribbon. This was necessary because molasses, one of the feed ingredients, stuck to them. The workers would scrape it down and wash it out. He and other employees were told to repeat the process several times because checks revealed continued contamination. According to *C*, the state officials made repeated checks of the plant, but the plant never was required to shut down. The plant suspended making feed for only one day, and that was in 1975.

The real hero of this story is a twenty-nine-year-old chemical-engineer-turned-dairy-farmer named Fred Halbert. As early as September 1973, Halbert noticed a decrease in milk production from his herd and unexplained deaths of some of his cows. He called in his veterinarian as well as experts from Michigan State University and officials from the Michigan Department of Agriculture. The experts could not diagnose the problem, and unfortunately the Michigan Department of Agriculture decided that there was no reason to curtail the sale of Halbert's milk. The MDA reasoned that, since no diagnosis could be made, it must be all right for humans to eat the sick animals and their products. Their decision resulted in the continued exposure of millions of Michigan residents to Firemaster.

Halbert noted that the onset of the illness and decreased milk production began shortly after he had been supplied with a new type of feed from the Michigan Farm Bureau Services, which supplied about one-third of Michigan's dairy farmers. He called the company, and they checked the feed but could find nothing wrong with it.

Having received no satisfaction thus far, Halbert started taking matters into his own hands. He set up his own feeding experiments and noted that the cows on the Michigan Farm Bureau feed became ill while cows on other feed did not. He then asked scientists with the Michigan Department of Agriculture to perform experiments with the cattle feed. Two groups of mice were fed the Farm Bureau feed, and all the mice in both groups were dead within two weeks! Still, no action was taken to withdraw the milk from human consumption.

By January 1974 Halbert had convinced Farm Bureau officials that something might be wrong with the feed. That month, Halbert noted that about half the calves produced in his herd were stillborn. He continued to press for an answer to the problem. Independent of state bureaucrats and company officials, he contacted scientists around the country at his own expense.

In April 1974 he finally received a break when he contacted Dr. George Fries, a chemist at the United States Department of Agriculture (USDA) Laboratory in Beltsville, Maryland. About this time, scientists with the U.S. Department of Agriculture at Ames, Iowa, who also were working on the problem, identified a bromine compound in the feed. Halbert passed this information on to Fries, who then, by mass spectroscopy, identified the compound as hexabromobiphenyl. The compound was traced back to the Michigan Chemical Corporation, which sells the material as Firemaster. Fries learned that Michigan Chemical had been supplying the Farm Bureau with another of its products, magnesium oxide, under the brand name Nutramaster. The answer then stuck out like a sore thumb. Michigan Chemical had sent the wrong product to the Farm Bureau.

A check of the Michigan Farm Bureau feed-mixing plant revealed numerous bags of Firemaster, stored, waiting to be mixed with cattle feed.

About mid-May 1974 articles began to appear in the *Detroit Free Press* concerning dairy herds contaminated with the bromine-containing flame retardant. I followed the stories with interest as the problem began to unfold in detail. The following account appeared in the May 29, 1974, edition of the *Free Press:*

MORE HERDS CONTAMINATED
AID ASKED FOR DAIRY FARMERS
By David Johnston

Lansing—State Agriculture Department inspectors reported
Tuesday finding traces of a deadly bromine compound in milk
from five additional dairy herds.

A total of 27 dairy herds and three beef cattle herds are
now known to have eaten Farm Bureau Services feeds contaminated with the substance intended for use as a fire retardant.

One of the dairymen sold his animals for slaughter last
January.

The article went on to review the previous findings. It was
now clear that this was an environmental contamination of major
proportions, with thousands, perhaps millions, of Michigan
residents exposed to the chemical through eating meat and dairy
products.

On May 28, 1974, one day before publication of the cited
Free Press story, I called the Michigan Chemical Corporation to
obtain a full description and a sample of the Firemaster product.
I asked about toxicity of the chemical and was informed that
thorough embryotoxicity, teratogenicity, and carcinogenicity
studies had not been performed on the product. I called Dr.
Benjamin Van Duuren, a leading chemical carcinogenesis expert
in New York, to inform him of the problem and to ask his advice.
He was especially concerned about possible product contaminants, such as dibenzofurans, that might be present, as well as
about the possible carcinogenicity of the polybrominated biphenyls themselves. Dibenzofurans are extremely toxic at levels as low
as several parts per billion. Certain contaminants could cause
cancer as well as birth defects.

That information made the problem even more devasting.
As far as I could determine, no one was planning to perform the
now very crucial toxicity studies on Firemaster. Since I had been
performing teratogenicity and carcinogenicity studies with inhalation anesthetic agents, I felt obligated to also perform these
studies on the polybrominated biphenyls.

Shortly after the discovery of Firemaster in the livestock

products, the FDA set a tolerance limit of 1 ppm of the chemical in the fat of animals. There was no scientific basis for the contention that 1 ppm is safe for human consumption. I was somewhat disturbed by this action on the part of the FDA.

Not much data were available on Firemaster, and what was known was hard to obtain. David Johnston, the reporter for the *Free Press* who had broken the story, had obtained a copy of a report from Michigan Chemical to the Michigan Environmental Review Board regarding Firemaster. He was kind enough to send a copy of the report to me.

The report was dated September 23, 1974. It stated that Firemaster BP-6 was a mixture of brominated biphenyls with an average bromine content equivalent to about six bromine atoms per biphenyl molecule. The product was said to be a mixture of the following brominated biphenyls:

Tetrabromobiphenyl	2.0%
Pentabromobiphenyl	10.6%
Hexabromobiphenyl	62.8%
Heptabromobiphenyl	13.8%
Other bromobiphenyls	11.4%

The report also stated that Firemaster is relatively inert chemically. It decomposes at temperatures of 300 to 400 degrees Centigrade. Firemaster effectively reduces the flammability of several thermoplastics, resulting in safer end-use products. Hexabromobiphenyl was, to the company's knowledge, the only polybrominated biphenyl manufactured and used on a commercial scale. E. I. duPont de Nemours & Company once considered using polybrominated biphenyls in the manufacture of flame retardant clothing, but decided against the idea after discovering that the compounds caused liver enlargement in rats.

Firemaster is used in the following products: typewriters, calculators, and microfilm reader housings, business machine housings, radio and television parts, thermostats, shaver and hand-tool housings, movie equipment cases, and miscellaneous small automotive parts.

The report also stated that Firemaster has been restricted to those applications where the end-use products were not exposed to either feed or food. Also, it is not used in flame-retardant fabrics to which humans would be exposed.

To the best of Michigan Chemical's knowledge, it was the only producer of polybrominated biphenyls in commercial quantity, and its yearly production was as follows:

1971	200,000 lbs.
1972	2,300,000 lbs.
1973	3,900,000 lbs.
1974 (projected)	4,800,000 lbs.

The report mentioned several studies of the acute toxicity of the product and one study of embryotoxicity. In the latter, birth defects were studied in rats, but the report neglected to state what abnormalities occurred. No carcinogenicity studies were mentioned.

The problem became more personal to me one weekend in July 1974 when I traveled north with my family to visit my brother and his wife near Traverse City. We had ordered animals for the PBB experiments earlier that week, and this was our last free weekend for a while.

My brother and his wife were renting a house on a farm. A friend who raised chickens had given them several of the birds as a present. My brother and sister-in-law were very pleased to be supplied with all the fresh eggs they could eat and took it as a personal affront when, after they proudly displayed their chickens, I commented that they were the most miserable-looking creatures I had ever seen. They were scrawny, and their feathers were falling out. They looked as if they had been half plucked. One had either a hernia or a tumor.

I asked what kind of feed they were eating, and my brother showed me a bag of Purina chicken feed. I said I believed the chickens had eaten PBB contaminated food sometime in the past. (By this time it was known that some chicken feed had been contaminated with PBB.) My brother called the woman who had given them the chickens, and sure enough, they had been given feed from the Michigan Farm Bureau Services! I advised my brother and his wife not to eat the eggs, at least until I had a chance to have several of them analyzed back in Ann Arbor.

I took some eggs that my brother gave me before we left (an act unknown to my sister-in-law, who was very attached to the chickens) to the Environmental Research Group in Ann Arbor for analysis. The results came back several days later: 0.06 parts PBB per million. It was there, all right—below the current tolerance, but still unsafe as far as I was concerned. (The tolerance for eggs later was lowered to 0.05 ppm.) My sister-in-law finally gave in and took the chickens to the humane society to be destroyed.

I soon learned what tremendous odds Fred Halbert had had to overcome to discover the etiology of his cows' illness. When I learned that the eggs from my brother and sister-in-law's chickens were contaminated with PBB, I assumed that all the eggs from the original flock of chickens also were contaminated. The woman who owned the flock had been selling eggs to stores around the Traverse City area. Her eggs were undoubtedly more highly contaminated than the ones I had tested because the chickens who had laid the tested eggs had not eaten the contaminated feed for about six weeks. The rest of the original flock probably was still eating it.

I started by calling the Michigan Department of Agriculture in Lansing. An official told me that it was ridiculous—no contaminated feed had been sent to the Traverse City area and the department was not going to check further into the matter; it was too far away. Besides, the levels in the eggs were within tolerance limits. My brother called the health department in Traverse City and a Michigan Department of Agriculture representative in his area. Both agencies refused to do anything. After several more calls, I finally gave up in disgust and advised my brother and his wife not to eat eggs. The rest of the population of Traverse City remained at risk by continuing to eat contaminated eggs. I did not know what else to do.

My experiment animals, pregnant mice, arrived and we were ready to go to work. Our research team consisted of myself, Dr. A. R. Beaudoin, professor of anatomy and a recognized expert on production of birth defects by chemicals, Dr. Richard G. Cornell, professor and chairman of the department of biostatistics, Judy Endres and Maria Swabodska, our technologists, and Bob Schumacher, a premedical student who was working with us for the summer. We prepared some rodent food spiced with 1,000 parts per million of the Firemaster compound. Judy, Maria, and

Bob took over the feeding of the animals after I instructed them in the proper handling of the Firemaster, which included wearing gloves and masks and mixing the food in a vented hood. We fed the experimental group from days seven through eighteen of the nineteen-day pregnancy period. The control group ate regular rodent food without the Firemaster.

We also began a preliminary carcinogenicity bioassay with Firemaster—a long-term study that was to last 15 months.

Several of the experimental animals died before the end of the feeding period. We performed autopsies on the animals and found two surprising things—the animals had died from massive gastrointestinal hemorrhages, and they all had greatly enlarged livers.

On day eighteen of the pregnancies, we killed the experimental and control animals with ether. Autopsies on the experimental animals revealed a continuing pattern of abnormal liver enlargement. We counted the number of dead fetuses. There were no major differences between the groups. There was some difference in the weights of the fetuses; the experimental fetuses weighed less than the controls. Bob, the premedical student, was opening the animals' abdomens, and Judy and Maria were weighing and preserving the fetuses. Suddenly Bob called out, "Look at this one!" We all looked at the strange-looking fetus he had discovered. The head was severely deformed, its brain protruding from the front and top of the skull.

"It's an exencephaly," I told them. "At least I'm pretty sure it is." I had never seen an exencephaly before, although I had read about them. We were all rather excited. An exencephaly could happen by chance, but we had never seen this deformity in the hundreds of mice we had examined in previous experiments. If it was due to the Firemaster, we would very likely see more of them in the remaining experimental animals.

Suddenly, Bob found another one. I was becoming convinced now. One exencephaly might have been just a fluke of nature, but two, although still not statistically significant, made me believe that we were on to something.

We ordered more pregnant mice and repeated the experiments, using 100 and 50 parts per million of Firemaster in the food. We also ran additional control groups. We found three more exencephalies in the group fed 100 ppm. Several weeks later, we examined the preserved fetuses for internal abnormalities and found four cleft palates in the group fed 1,000 ppm and one in the group fed 50 ppm. None appeared in the controls. This data further suggested that something in the Firemaster compound was weakly teratogenic.

Just before we began our teratogenicity studies with Firemaster, an article appeared in the *Ann Arbor News* about the Environmental Research Group, a private laboratory in Ann Arbor that was measuring the amounts of Firemaster in food products for the Michigan Farm Bureau Services. I called the laboratory and talked with Dr. Frank Hammer, an analytical chemist with the firm. We decided to study tissue levels of PBB in some of our animals to confirm that the experimental mice had indeed eaten the Firemaster during the course of the experiment. We also decided to study the levels of polybrominated biphenyls in human fat samples taken from randomly selected autopsies. We later studied fat specimens from three nonfarm residents of Michigan and found detectable levels of polybrominated biphenyls in all three.

In September 1974 I attended a meeting at the Michigan Farm Bureau in Lansing. The meeting was attended by members of the Farm Bureau, dairy farmers, scientists, attorneys, representatives of the Michigan Chemical Corporation, representatives of involved insurance companies, and officials of the Michigan Department of Agriculture. The purpose of the meeting was to discuss what to do about the thousands of dairy cows that were producing milk contaminated with PBB, but below the current tolerance level of 1 ppm.

Dairy farmers told of cows that were currently running low levels of PBB but showed symptoms such as weight loss, swollen joints, decreased milk production, and skin sores. They expressed concern about selling the milk from these cows for human consumption. I, too, was concerned that the FDA had set the tolerance so high with no proof whatsoever that 1 ppm was a safe concentration.

Dr. Fries, the chemist from the U.S. Department of Agriculture, told of studies of the half-life of polybrominated biphenyls in animals. It had been thought that if the cows were kept long enough perhaps the PBB levels would drop below tolerance so that milk could again be sold and the cows eventually slaughtered and sold for human consumption. According to the studies presented by Fries, it would be a poor gamble at best.

The major concern seemed to be the economic loss (which was staggering) and how to get out of this mess as inexpensively as possible. No one mentioned the possible harm to the human population that had been so widely exposed until I raised the question. I said that our primary concern must be for the health and welfare of the people of Michigan. I expressed my concern that the tolerance level had been set too high without evidence that the level was really safe. I then asked Fries if the material had been analyzed for impurities. He said that it had not. I stated that under the circumstances, they were totally ignorant of the potential damage to the human population from this material. Firemaster could contain a number of different impurities with devastating toxicity. Determination of the contents of Firemaster should have been the first priority so we would at least know to what chemicals the population had been exposed. I mentioned the possibility that Firemaster could be a material like the herbicide 2,4,5-T, in which the dioxin contaminant was the real problem, not the herbicide itself. We were dealing with a material which had not been fully analyzed.

We then went outside the building to see two calves that one of the dairy farmers had brought to the meeting. They were pitiful-looking animals, small for their ages, and covered with scales and sores. The farmer mentioned that he had been going to bring another calf that looked even worse, but it had died the night before.

When the meeting resumed, I presented my group's data on the birth defects produced in mice with Firemaster, emphasizing that some component of the product appeared to be producing the defects. I stated that certain chemicals that were known to produce birth defects in animals also were carcinogenic, and this possibility must also be considered with Firemaster. I also mentioned the large livers we had seen in the experimental animals. I restated my position that I did not feel that a tolerance of 1 ppm in food for human consumption was safe.

The farmers were excused after the first part of the meeting, but first each one was offered the opportunity to convey his thoughts about the situation, particularly his feelings about destroying cows that had low levels of contamination. These farmers were men who, through no fault of their own, had been subjected to a year of uncertainty, unhappiness, financial disaster, heartache, and at times, guilt. They all expressed their concern about selling contaminated products to consumers. One of the men told that after seeing his cows looking so ill, even though the tests showed the PBB levels to be below tolerance, he had stopped drinking milk from his own cows and bought milk for his family at the grocery store. It tasted "lousy," he said, but they were getting used to it.

Then a young man in his mid-twenties rose slowly from his chair. He began to speak, his voice cracking slightly.

"We'll do whatever you decide about the animals. I—I just—" His voice was quivering. "I just want to—to get it over with so we can have a normal life again. It's been so hard on—It's—"

"It's enough to make a grown man sit and cry," I thought to myself, the words of the song by John Denver echoed through my mind as I watched the young man, with tears rolling down his cheeks, sit down and bury his head in his arms.

The meeting at the Michigan Farm Bureau seemed to stimulate some activity. Dr. George Whitehead, deputy director of the Michigan Department of Agriculture, decided on the basis of the discussions to organize a meeting with members of the Food and Drug Administration. This meeting was held in Lansing on October 9, 1974. By this time we had amassed more data from our studies, and I was asked to present it.

Three officials from the Food and Drug Administration attended, along with representatives of the Michigan Department of Agriculture, researchers from Michigan State University, veterinarians, a state senator, and several dairy farmers, including Fred Halbert.

I presented our findings, including the human PBB levels, slides of the animals with birth defects and liver changes. I again expressed my concern for the exposed human population in terms of cancer production and birth defects in offspring.

Further progress followed this meeting. The FDA asked for copies of our report, and several weeks later FDA officials made a field trip to examine cows that were producing milk below tolerance but still appeared ill. Subsequently, on November 4, 1974, they lowered the tolerance limit from 1 ppm to 0.3 ppm in meat and poultry, and to 0.05 ppm in eggs. This ruling resulted in the eventual destruction of about 20,000 more cows and increased protection of the people of Michigan from the ingestion of polybrominated biphenyls.

It was gratifying to know that our work had been somewhat instrumental in bringing about this change. However, I was not convinced that the new tolerance levels were safe. Furthermore, Firemaster had not yet been thoroughly analyzed for impurities.

In October 1974 I called Dr. Irving Selikoff, Professor of Environmental Medicine, Mount Sinai School of Medicine, and requested his assistance in the matter. He was very concerned and offered the assistance of his staff and laboratory. On October 29, 1974, a member of his staff, Dr. Henry Anderson, flew to Michigan to review the problem with me. I informed him of the details of the episode to that time. He returned to New York and conferred with Dr. Selikoff, who then offered to send a team of experts to Michigan to investigate the problem, all without charge to the state of Michigan. Dr. Selikoff informed me that he did not feel that he should begin the investigation without an official invitation from the state officials. I called Dr. George Whitehead of the Michigan Department of Agriculture and I also called Governor Milliken's office and informed both of Dr. Selikoff's expertise and interest in the problem. I told an aid to Governor Milliken that I felt the state agencies did not have the expertise to handle the PBB problem. I recommended that Dr. Selikoff be issued an invitation to investigate the problem.

Dr. Selikoff never received the invitation.

In the spring of 1975, it was learned that some farmers were selling both live and dead contaminated animals to rendering plants instead of disposing of them in an environmentally protective manner. Rendering plants process the dead animals into (believe it or not) livestock feed as well as dog and cat food. Other products include tallow and grease for soaps and shampoos. Scientists became concerned that this practice would lead to an endless cycle of PBB contamination in Michigan.

An article in the *Grand Rapids Press* quoted one farmer as saying, "I'm having the rendering plant pick up my cows." His farm was quarantined by the state after levels up to 1.6 ppm of the flame retardant chemical were found in his pigs. His cows also had measurable levels. The farmer said that he had sent for the trucks from the rendering plant because the Michigan Farm Bureau refused to take the cows. "It's crazy, though," the farmer said. "The renderer just grinds the animals up and sells them back to the farmer again."

Another farmer said that his cows had levels as high as 5,000 ppm. He estimated that he had sent at least fifty of these animals to the rendering plant before he was quarantined. "When the state first found the PBB in the cattle," he said, "it only warned the farmer. It did not quarantine him. So he could have taken dead ones to the renderer."

The manager of the Battle Creek rendering plant was contacted and told the *Grand Rapids Press* that there is no state check to determine whether his plant accepts animals contaminated with PBB. He also stated that the plant delivers its products to grain elevators across the state, including some run by the Michigan Farm Bureau.

A spokesman for another rendering plant said that his firm refuses to take quarantined animals, but one farmer who does business with this plant said that he was never questioned whether his animals were contaminated.

It was discovered that one farmer whose animals had measurable levels of PBB sent them to an Indiana rendering plant, which turned the cows into poultry feed and bone meal, while some of the byproducts were incorporated into medicines, buffing compounds, and shaving lotions.

State officials said they left the disposal of dead animals to the Michigan Farm Bureau Services, since they had no authority to do otherwise. A Michigan Department of Agriculture veterinarian told the *Grand Rapids Press* that the department had no authority to force farmers to save carcasses for burial at the state-designated site near Kalkaska, Michigan.

The Michigan Department of Natural Resources also stated that it had no authority over the burial of contaminated cattle. *The Grand Rapids Press* concluded:

> . . . The state's loose leadership in accounting for the dead cattle in what has been called the largest poisoning incident in the nation's history has brought about the spread, rather than the removal of, polybrominated biphenyls from the environment.

Farmers began filing suit against the Michigan Farm Bureau for selling contaminated livestock feed that resulted in the destruction of their livestock and their livelihood. By fall 1974 suits totaling over $100 million had been filed.

The Michigan Farm Bureau in turn filed a $277 million lawsuit against the Michigan Chemical Corporation, charging that Michigan Chemical had sent polybrominated biphenyls to it in place of the magnesium oxide that had been ordered. Other plaintiffs in the suit were Firemen's Fund Insurance Company and Auto-Owners Insurance Company, who insure Michigan Farm Bureau. Other defendants listed in the suit were Northwest Industries and the Michigan Salt Company.

At the time the lawsuit was filed, more than 9,000 cattle had been destroyed and buried at the Kalkaska burial site. In addition, 900,000 chickens, 1.5 million eggs, 2,200 pigs, 1,000 pheasants, 348 sheep, and 10,000 pounds of cheese also had been destroyed, and the toll continued to rise.

By the end of April 1975, 15,942 cattle, 3,469 pigs, 394 sheep, over 1 million chickens, and tons of eggs, milk, cheese, butter, and other products had been destroyed because they had been contaminated with polybrominated biphenyls.

None of the involved state agencies or the involved companies pursued my early recommendations to identify all the chemicals in Firemaster. Finally, in September 1975, Gary Schenk, an attorney from Grand Rapids representing farmers with affected animals, contacted Dr. Patrick O'Keefe of Harvard University's Department of Chemistry and aroused his interest in the problem. Dr. O'Keefe studied samples of Firemaster and by early November of that year he had identified polybrominated naphthalenes in the mixture. Subsequently, Dr. John A. Moore of the National Institute of Environmental Health Sciences reported finding a methyl polybrominated furan in Firemaster. These were extremely important findings because these compounds are most likely extremely toxic at very low concentrations. It is known that poly*chlorinated* naphthalenes and dibenzofurans are very toxic, and there is reason to suspect that the brominated counterparts are even more toxic than the chlorinated ones.

O'Keefe's initial findings were made known in January 1976. The presence of brominated naphthalenes in Firemaster did not appear to be of concern to the Michigan Department of Agriculture or the Department of Public Health.

Dairy farmer Gerry Woltjer of Coopersville, Michigan, had a herd of 300 cows. For the past year he had noticed them deteriorate: milk production was down, there was an increase in stillborn calves, and mature cows were dying. They developed enlarged hooves, swollen joints, and weight loss. Agriculture department officials blamed the problem on "mismanagement."

In February 1976 Woltjer had two sick cows tested for PBB and below tolerance concentrations were found in both animals. The animals had symptoms similar to high level PBB animals, yet they were below tolerance and Woltjer was not eligible for any type of assistance.

In April 1976, in desperation, Gerry Woltjer shot the 230 remaining cows in his herd.

Another dairy farmer, Louis Trombley of Hersey, Michigan, had similar problems with his animals. His animals had low concentrations of PBB, yet Trombley never bought feed from Farm Bureau Services. He just used Michigan Chemical salt. "I just couldn't see selling milk and meat with poison in 'em so as people could eat it, especially little kids," Trombley was quoted as saying. He also shot his cows.

Other farmers complained that animals were sick and dying. Cows were infertile and calves that were born had a high incidence of stillbirth and early mortality, as high as 50 percent on some farms. Other animals were dying, including birds, cats, mice, and rats. Some of these farmers never used Michigan Farm

Bureau products. The Michigan Department of Agriculture also blamed these deaths and this illness in cows on "mismanagement," although most of the involved farmers were experienced in dairy herd management. Furthermore, "mismanagement" did not explain the deaths of the other animals. In addition to the animals, the farmers and their families were noticing health problems, including skin rashes and acne-like lesions, fatigue, weight loss, joint and muscle pains, and menstrual disorders.

The lack of action on the part of state agencies was disturbing. In May 1976 attorney Gary Schenk invited Dr. Patrick O'Keefe and me to tour some of the affected farms. We were amazed to learn that dairy cows were still sick and dying, and their milk was still being sold for human consumption. The PBB levels of these cows were below tolerance. Apparently for this reason, the MDA condoned the sale of the milk and beef from these diseased animals.

It was a disturbing situation. These animals had low levels of PBB; however, many of the farms had never received cow feed from the Michigan Farm Bureau. One farmer who had received Farm Bureau feed told me that he had his milk tested only once. The MDA took six milk samples. Of these six samples, four were reported as "lost" and the other two were below tolerance. That test was in the spring of 1975. His animals were never tested again, even though he complained that they were sick and dying.

No one had investigated the possibility that the salt products might be contaminated. It appeared to be a possible explanation for some of the farmers' problems with their animals. Michigan Chemical produces their salt products on the same grounds as many of their toxic chemical products, including *Firemaster*. One farmer was so suspicious of this relationship that he sent salt samples to a laboratory for analysis. He produced a laboratory report showing the salt to be contaminated with low concentrations of not only polybrominated biphenyls, but poly*chlorinated* biphenyls and polychlorinated *terphenyls* as well! It is hard to believe that corporate officials would allow the production of toxic chemicals near food supplements, and that there are no federal regulations to prevent such an occurrence. But that is how it is. It is possible that the salt products from Michigan Chemical (which are shipped outside of Michigan as well) contain other contaminants in addition to the PBBs, PCBs, and PCTs.

By early May 1976 the death toll had reached 32,000 cows, 6,000 pigs, 1,370 sheep, and 1.5 million chickens. In addition, 18,000 pounds of cheese, 2,630 pounds of butter, and 34,000 pounds of dry milk products and 5 million eggs had been destroyed due to Firemaster contamination.

Farmers continued to complain that sick animals and their products were still reaching consumers and that state officials were still trying to "cover up" the incident, which they now referred to as "Cattlegate."

Agriculture Officiials contended that farmers were exaggerating the extent of the PBB contamination and were using it as an excuse for poor livestock management.

In early 1976, Governor William Milliken appointed a panel of scientists to study the PBB problem and make recommendations concerning the current tolerance limits for the chemicals in food for human consumption. Dr. Isodore Bernstein, professor of biological chemistry and environmental and industrial health at the University of Michigan, was chairman of the advisory panel. A second wise choice was Dr. Benjamin Van Duuren (see Chapters 3 and 14). However, three of the original five members were not wisely chosen. One initially declined because of a conflict of interest. He was employed by a major chemical company. The fourth member of the original panel had been given money to study Firemaster by the Michigan Chemical Company and the the fifth member of the panel expressed concern that the fourth might be biased on that basis. The fourth member was asked to leave. The fifth member was then asked to leave for unknown reasons. Four additional members were then chosen and the panel began its study and deliberations.

The panel met with scientists involved in research related to the problem and with members of the Michigan Department of Agriculture. I was asked to present my findings to the panel on April 19, 1976, at the Hilton Inn, Detroit Metropolitan Airport, and I began my testimony by discussing the birth defects studies I had performed in 1974 and expressing my concern at the time that dibenzofurans or other contaminants might be present in Firemaster. I stated that I also started a preliminary carcinogenicity bioassay with Firemaster and gave the panel the following summary of that investigation, stating that it was to be considered preliminary in nature, but the results considerably heightened my suspicions of the carcinogenicity of one or more of the components of Firemaster.

> Six timed-pregnant Swiss/ICR mice were fed 100 ppm Firemaster in rodent chow from days 7–18 of the pregnancy. Six identical mice were fed normal rodent chow as controls. The animals were allowed to deliver spontaneously. The offspring were nursed by their mothers and maintained for 15 months. Mothers were also allowed to live the additional 15 months.
>
> Five of the six mothers fed Firemaster died prior to the termination of the experiment. Because of inadequate personnel in the animal facilities, we were not notified of the deaths of these animals and they were not examined. At the time of autopsy, the one remaining mother had multiple tumors throughout the liver. The hexabromobiphenyl concentration in this liver was 2.4 ppm. 1/22 male offspring had a solitary nodule on the liver. 0/20 female offspring had tumors. None of the control animals had tumors. The tumors from both the experimental mother and offspring were examined histologically by Dr. Hans Popper, Mt. Sinai Medical Center, New York. A copy of his report is attached.

I then explained the principles of chemical carcinogenesis for those members of the panel who were not involved in this specific type of research. I then expressed my concern over Dr. O'Keefe's discover of polybrominated naphthalenes in Firemaster. I showed a chart comparing the symptoms seen in cows poisoned with poly*chlorinated* naphthalenes (see Chapter 9—"X" disease) and the symptoms seen in the Firemaster cows. The symptoms were almost identical. In addition, many of the symptoms seen in people exposed to chlorinated naphthalenes were similar to the complaints expressed by Michigan farmers and their families. I ended my testimony by stating that research in animals suggests that compounds such as dibenzofurans, dioxins and naphthalenes appear to have cumulative toxicity, and the risk of continued long-term exposure is great.

Other scientists who testified before the panel include Dr.

Irving Selikoff, Professor of Environmental Medicine, Mount Sinai School of Medicine (see Chapters 3, 12, and 14), and Dr. James R. Allen, University of Wisconsin Primate Research Center (see Chapter 9).

On May 24, 1976, the panel and Governor Milliken announced the panel's recommendations. The panel unanimously recommended that the state lower the level of acceptable amounts of PBB in food for human consumption immediately because of concern over the possible long-term cumulative effects on human health. The panel recommended that the current guidelines set by the U.S. Food and Drug Administration at 0.3 ppm for meat be lowered to 0.005 ppm, and the guidelines for milk be lowered to 0.001 ppm. The panel made further recommendations, including long-term follow-up of exposed individuals and the institution of safeguards to prevent another similar disaster in the future.

One would think that the Michigan Department of Agriculture would adopt the panel's recommendation with all due haste, and the chain of ignorance and stupidity which allowed the Firemaster incident to occur and continue would be broken. Unfortunately, such was not the case.

On June 10, 1976, the Michigan Department of Agriculture held a public hearing in Lansing, to hear testimony concerning the reduction of permissible tolerance for polybrominated biphenyls as recommended by the governor's scientific panel. There was a well-organized program representing industry and others with interests in not lowering the tolerance. In addition, an official of the Food and Drug Administraiton (an organization with a reputation for slowness in reacting to suspicious chemicals in foods, viz., Red No. 2, diethylstilbestrol, etc.) stated that the FDA saw no reason to change the tolerance.

When my turn came to testify, I made the following statement:

> "The Firemaster incident is now an environmental contamination episode of monumental proportions. Let us reflect for a few moments on the events which allowed it to occur and be perpetuated for so long.
>
> It started at the Michigan Chemical Company, which makes a variety of toxic chemical products in close proximity to salt

products which are used as supplements for livestock feed. The company chose similar brand names for two of their products— one a toxic chemical mixture, the other a salt supplement for livestock. Sometime in early 1973, Michigan Chemical stopped using well-marked bags for these products and switched to plain brown bags with only the brand name stencilled on it. *Firemaster,* the toxic chemical mixture, was sent to Michigan Farm Bureau mixing plants instead of Nutramaster, the magnesium oxide supplement.

Now let us switch our attention to the Michigan Farm Bureau. Although the bags were labelled with a brand name for a product not previously used by the Farm Bureau, the mistake was not discovered. *Firemaster* was mixed with livestock feed and shipped to farmers around the state.

Farmers began to complain that animals were sick and milk production was decreased. The Michigan Department of Agriculture was not able to diagnose the problem. Instead of curtailing the sale of animals and their products, as common sense would dictate, the Michigan Department of Agriculture permitted the sale of these sick animals and their products, thus exposing millions of consumers throughout the state to *Firemaster.* The illness among dairy cows was first reported about September, 1973. About January, 1974, the Michigan Department of Agriculture reportedly conducted a feeding experiment using livestock feed from a farm with sick animals. Two groups of mice were fed the livestock feed, and within two weeks every mouse in both groups was dead. Still nothing was done to stop the sale of sick animals or their products for human consumption. Furthermore, it was through the valiant efforts of an individual farmer that the true nature of the livestock illness was discovered, not through the efforts of our regulatory agencies.

It was not until April, 1974, that *Firemaster* was found to be the toxic contaminant in the livestock feed. Without any proof that the level was safe, the Food and Drug Administration set a tolerance limit of 1 part per million on a fat basis in food for human consumption. The FDA based this level on what officials said was the current limit of detection in the laboratory, when in fact other laboratories were measuring concentrations considerably below that level. After later consideration the tolerance was reduced to 0.3 parts per million.

Shortly after *Firemaster* was discovered in the livestock feed, I expressed my concern, both to officials and publicly, that *Firemaster* most likely contained highly toxic contaminants, and that *Firemaster* must be considered as highly suspicious in terms of causing long-term human illness, specifically birth defects and cancer. My warnings were ignored.

It was later found that *Firemaster* does indeed contain contaminants which are suspected to be highly toxic. Again, it was not our regulatory agencies which made the discovery. These findings were made through the efforts of an attorney and a veterinarian who contacted a Harvard University scientist and interested him in the problem. The scientist in turn made the discovery.

Once animals were quarantined, disposal of these animals was poorly controlled. Animals were sold to rendering plants which ground up the carcasses and sold parts of them back to farmers as more livestock feed, thus further spreading the contamination.

Thus, for three years, the people of the state of Michigan have been eating food contaminated with a mixture of chemicals suspected of causing long term, or delayed onset, disease conditions.

Now a panel of six eminent scientists has studied the problem and made recommendations. They have concluded that the long-term risks of continued exposure to *Firemaster* are too great to take, and human consumption should be reduced to the lowest measurable concentration. The panel has studied the analytical methods available and those currently employed, and concluded that the minimum detectable level should be 5 parts per *billion* for meat and 1 part per *billion* for milk. The panel further recommended that these action guidelines be constantly reviewed to determine whether they can be lowered even further with improving technology.

These recommendations were made unanimously by six eminent scientists with expertise in the appropriate subjects, including chemical carcinogenesis. These are intelligent, highly knowledgable, and honest men. I see no further reason to debate their recommendations.

If the Michigan Department of Agriculture feels that it cannot currently meet the panel's recommended guidelines, it should request the appropriate funds from the legislature to equip their laboratories with the instrumentation and technicians necessary to meet these standards.

Implementation of the panel's recommendations will be costly. However, the cost of a major disease epidemic in the state of Michigan will be far costlier. Being entrusted with protecting the health and welfare of the people of the state of Michigan is an awesome responsibility, and I remind our public officials that the people of the state of Michigan, who place you in your offices either directly or indirectly, take the panel's recommendations very seriously. They want untainted food for themselves and especially for their children.

We are past the point where we can allow industry, lobbyists, and politicians to decide what our levels of exposure to toxic chemicals will be. It is time to listen to the scientists who know the truth regarding the tremendous consequences we may face unless rather extreme measure are implemented soon. Otherwise we, and more tragically, our children and their children, will have to pay the ultimate consequences for our ignorance and our stupidity."

Two weeks later the Michigan Department of Agriculture announced its decision. It totally rejected the recommendations of Governor Milliken's scientific advisory panel by refusing to lower the tolerance by any amount. Thus, the people of Michigan continue to eat *Firemaster*.

In mid-1976 the Michigan Department of Public Health announced the results of a study of PBB levels in human breast milk. Sixteen mothers from Michigan's lower peninsula were tested and all sixteen had measurable concentrations of the chemical in their milk. In addiition, six of ten women from Michigan's upper peninsula also had measurable levels. These findings reflect the massive contamination of the food supply and suggest that the great majority of Michigan consumers now have PBBs stored in their body tissues.

Another disturbing finding was announced in September 1976. Five people poisoned in the Yusho incident with the related chemicals, PCBs, had developed liver cancer. This is fifteen times the expected rate for that given group of people. Both PCBs and PBBs had been suspected of causing liver cancer—at least for PCBs, this now appears to be a fact.

The Firemaster incident is now the worst single environmental contamination episode in history. Had the incident been investigated by competent people initially, the contaminant and its source would have been identified and eliminated in the fall of 1973. The ignorance and stupidity which caused the incident and allowed it to continue must be remembered, or it will happen again.

11
Minamata

The problems of overpopulation and industrialization are tragically evident to the 108 million people in Japan, where over 100 people have died in one town as a result of the local chemical plant's pouring wastes into local waters. The town is Minamata, and it has the dubious distinction of having the disease caused by the pollution named after it—Minamata disease.

Minamata is a Japanese fishing and farming village on the island of Kyushu. Its people joined the industrial age in .1907 when a factory was built there. The company later became known as the Chisso Corporation. Chisso (which means "nitrogen" in Japanese) began as a carbide and fertilizer company and has grown into a major petrochemical and plastics producer.

By 1925 wastes from Chisso had already damaged fishing areas in Minamata Bay and was paying a small indemnity to local fishermen. In 1932 Chisso began production of the chemical acetaldehyde, used in a number of industrial processes including the manufacture of plastics, drugs, photographic chemicals, and perfume. The chemical process for making acetaldehyde requires the use of a mercury compound as a catalyst. By 1950 the production of acetaldehyde had increased dramatically because of its use in the manufacture of the plasticizer dioctyl phthalate.

Chisso continued to pour its wastes, including mercury, through pipes into Minamata Bay. Over the years the bay became a sludge dump for a variety of chemicals.

As the chemicals increased in concentration in the bay they also accumulated in the fish. The mercury became incorporated into microorganisms as the organic compound methyl mercury. The microorganisms were then ingested by the fish, which became progressively poisoned. The fishermen of Minamata continued fishing, and the fish ended up on the dinner tables of the residents. For many of the town's inhabitants, fish constituted the bulk of their diet.

As the years passed, fish catches became smaller. Dead fish were noticed floating on the surface of the water, victims of the pollution. The number of shellfish diminished. By 1952 crows and sea birds began dropping dead into the sea while flying. Even seaweed died.

People who ate large quantities of the fish began to manifest symptoms of an unknown illness. They called it the "strange disease." The residents also noticed that cats were afflicted with what they called "dancing disease." The animals would stagger as if drunk. They would salivate excessively and suddenly go into convulsions or whirl in violent circles and finally collapse. Others went similarly berserk, falling into the sea as though they were committing suicide. The cats started having "dancing disease" in the early 1950s, and by 1958 there were virtually no cats left in certain areas of Minamata. Other animals were afflicted with the disease, including dogs and pigs.

The first definite case of Minamata disease in humans was reported in 1953, although it later became obvious that earlier deaths, at the time unrecognized, had occurred. In April 1956 a five-year-old girl was admitted to the Chisso Corporation's Minamata factory hospital with symptoms of brain damage, including disturbances of speech and gait. She was delirious. About a month later her younger sister and four members of a neighboring family were found to be suffering similar symptoms. On the first of May, 1956, Dr. Hajimé Hosokawa, head of the

Chisso hospital, reported that an undiagnosed disease of the central nervous system had broken out. This was the official "discovery" of what was later to be called Minamata disease.

An investigation quickly uncovered thirty more cases in the area. The first symptoms had developed in these people around 1953. The outbreak was treated as an epidemic of an infectious disease because the true cause was unknown. In August 1956 a research group from the Kumamoto University Medical School was created to investigate the disease. By October the group issued an interim report that the epidemic was not infectious, but was caused by a type of heavy metal poisoning from eating the fish and shellfish of Minamata Bay.

The logical measures to take at this point would have included banning fishing in the area and shutting the Chisso plant until the type of heavy metal poisoning was determined and alternate methods of disposing of the offending substance were developed. Neither measure was taken. Fishing continued and Chisso continued polluting the bay with chemical wastes. By the end of 1956 there were fifty-two reported patients with Minamata disease.

The research group continued its studies. It learned that the Chisso wastes included manganese, arsenic, copper, lead, selenium, mercury, and thallium. It conducted experiments on each poison. At first the most highly suspect of these were manganese, selenium, and thallium. Large quantities of each were found in patients at autopsy and large amounts also were found in the environment. None of the three, however, produced the symptoms seen in animals or people.

In other experiments fish were brought into the bay from outside areas and were found to accumulate heavy metals rapidly. When these fish were then fed to cats, the cats developed symptoms of "dancing disease." This showed the magnitude of the contamination in the bay. In another experiment imported cats were fed fish from Minamata Bay, and they developed symptoms of the illness after eating the fish for as short a time as thirty-two days.

Finally, in September 1958, one of the researchers discovered that the symptoms and pathological findings in cases of Minamata disease were similar to those of methyl mercury poisoning reported in workers at a plant producing the chemical in England in 1940. The researchers then experimented by feeding methyl mercury to cats. The animals developed the same symptoms as the cats in Minamata. Researchers then studied the Minamata environment for the presence of methyl mercury. In 1959 it was found that methyl mercury was present in the remarkably high concentration of 2,010 parts per million in the mud of the drainage channels of the Chisso plant. Fish and shellfish collected from the bay had levels as high as 39 ppm. Mercury levels in both experimental and local cats were found to be as high as 145 ppm in liver, 36 ppm in kidneys, 18 ppm in brain, and even 70 ppm in hair.

It was later discovered that methyl mercury is formed from inorganic mercury compounds by microorganisms living in river and lake bottom deposits. In an experiment that proved this theory, samples of bottom sediment were treated with 100 ppm mercuric chloride (an inorganic compound) and allowed to stand for five or ten days. The levels of methyl mercury (an organic compound) rose progressively with time. If the bottom sediment were sterilized first, killing the microorganisms, no methyl mercury was formed. If the sterilized samples were then reinoculated with the microorganisms and the experiment repeated, the methyl mercury levels again rose with time.

Chisso used large quantities of mercury in both the acetaldehyde and vinyl chloride manufacturing processes. Estimates of the total amount of mercury dumped into Minamata Bay by Chisso ranged from 200 to 600 tons.

Detailed examination of patients with Minamata disease revealed that the symptoms started with numbness of the extremities and lips, difficulty in grasping things with the hands, lack of coordination, weakness, and tremor. Damage to the cerebellum resulted in speech disturbances. Patients would lose the ability to walk straight and then develop visual disturbances and impaired hearing. These symptoms would gradually increase in severity, leading to paralysis, deformity, difficulty in swallowing, convulsions, and finally death. These symptoms are indicative of damage to the nervous system. Autopsies on patients dying of Minamata disease revealed damage to cells in various parts of the brain and other parts of the nervous system. Concentrations of mercury were measured in patients who died. The greatest concentrations were found in the liver and kidneys, up to 70 ppm and 144 ppm respectively. Brains had concentrations up to 21 ppm. Later studies revealed that hair especially concentrated the chemical. Concentrations as high as 700 ppm have been reported.

By the end of 1962 there were 121 proven cases of Minamata disease, and 46 of the victims had died.

Several cases of congenital idiocy with serious disturbances of coordination, tremors, growth disturbances, deformities, and other symptoms had been reported in the Minamata area about the same time as the onset of Minamata disease. Autopsies of several affected children who died revealed degenerative and regressive changes in the cells of the cerebral cortex. The one common factor in these cases was that the mother had eaten large quantities of fish and shellfish from the bay during pregnancy.

Between 1955 and 1958, 220 births occurred in the areas of the town hardest hit by Minamata disease. Among the 220 infants there were 13 cases of idiocy—almost 6 percent. Sixty-four percent of these affected children were born into families in which a member had Minamata disease. Careful examination of the mothers of these children revealed that in 73 percent of the cases, the mothers had early or mild symptoms of methyl mercury poisoning. By 1962 two of the afflicted children had died. The post-mortem examinations revealed typical indications of methyl mercury poisoning. It was clear that these were cases of congenital Minamata disease. The chemical had passed across the placenta from the mother to the fetus and affected it during development. By 1974 forty cases of congenital methyl mercury poisoning were diagnosed in the Minamata area.

Mercury compounds have been shown to cause both fetal death and birth defects in several animals. Mice given high doses of a mercury compound (ethylmercuric phosphate) intravenously on day ten of the pregnancy produced a high incidence of cleft palate in the offspring. Another mercury compound (methyl mercury dicyaniamide) injected into the abdomen on day ten resulted in a significant increase in fetal mortality. In another experiment rats given a single oral dose of 2 milligrams of methyl mercury chloride on day nine, ten, or eleven of the twenty-one-day pregnancy produced offspring with brain defects, including distortion of the shape of the entire cerebellum, enlarged ventricular cavities, and degeneration of nerve cells. Small doses (0.2 milligrams per day) given throughout the pregnancy resulted in a number of microscopic changes in brain cells present both at birth and when the babies reached maturity. The changes in the brain cells were similar to those seen in Minamata disease. Similar findings have also been demonstrated in cats. Thus, experiments have demonstrated that mercury can produce fetal death and birth defects in mice, rats, and cats.

From these experiments it appears that fetal tissue, especially nervous tissue, is damaged by low concentrations of mercury. This also appears to be true in the human, and it is likely that the safe level for the pregnant human temale is extremely low.

In December 1959 Chisso installed a device called a cyclator to process its waste material. The public was told that the device would remove the mercury from the waste before dumping it into the bay.

It was later discovered that the device was not effective, and the mercury continued to pour into the waters around Minamata. By 1962 it was generally believed that the problem was over and people again began to eat large quantities of fish from the bay without reservation.

The pollution continued. The Chisso Corporation did nothing. The government did not conduct or sponsor research into the problem, nor did it impose any ban on fishing in the area. The fishermen, being dependent on the fish for their livelihood and diet, kept quiet. Many people were afraid to be examined due to the social stigma that became attached to having the disease. Many mild cases of methyl mercury poisoning went unreported.

Finally, in 1970, medical researchers surveyed the population and discovered many cases previously unreported. Eighty-four percent of the family members of patients with the established diagnosis of Mimanata disease were found to have symptoms of the disease themselves. Mothers of infants with the congenital form of the disease all suffered from mild symptoms. Surveys of the general population in areas of the town hardest hit revealed symptoms in a large number of the people. Twenty-eight percent of the people had sensory disturbances; 24 percent had problems with coordination; 29 percent had hearing problems; 13 percent had constricted visual fields; and tremors were found in 10 percent.

By 1974 there were 798 patients with verified cases of Minamata disease; 107 of these had died. Another 2,800 inhabitants of the area had applied for examination and verification.

The symptoms of Minamata disease depend on the concentration of methyl mercury to which the victim is exposed and the length of time over which it is ingested. After a high-dose ingestion, the victim has symptoms of acute brain damage, including disturbance of consciousness, convulsions, paralysis, and finally death. With intake of lower concentrations the symptoms are slower in onset and not as rapidly fatal. With even lower concentrations the onset is slower yet, and the symptoms may be such nonspecific conditions as high blood pressure or hepatitis.

The predominant effect of methyl mercury poisoning is the central nervous system, but other organs are affected too. There is evidence that the chemical may, as just mentioned, cause high blood pressure and liver damage, and in addition, cause diabetes. Autopsies of patients have shown damage to kidneys, liver, pancreas, and bone marrow.

The effect of methyl mercury on the fertile female also varies with the dose. An acute high dose leads to infertility. If the dosage if less, pregnancy may occur, but the fetus will be either aborted or stillborn. If the dose is somewhat lower, the child will be born alive, but with severe congenital Minamata disease. A still lower dose will result in a child that is only somewhat mentally retarded with few or no other symptoms. A study revealed that 29 percent of the children born in the areas with the highest incidence of the disease between 1955 and 1959 were mentally deficient. Furthermore, a study of junior high school students in these areas made in 1970 revealed that 21 percent of the children had sensory disturbances; 18 percent were mentally dificient; and 12 percent had speech impediments.

The pattern of events in the Minamata incident is astounding in terms of the total lack of regard for those affected. For years, industry apparently tried to sweep the whole problem under the rug, denying its role in the poisoning while letting it continue. Nor did the government control the situation. It would have been simple to shut down the Chisso plant and ban fishing in the area. Neither was done. It was only after the problem became blatant that any studies were initiated, and these were conducted by independent researchers.

Minamata should be a good history lesson for all of us. We cannot afford to discard the lessons of the past.

Minamata was not the only Japanese city to be hit with methyl mercury poisoning. There was an outbreak in 1966 in the city of Niigata, hundreds of miles from Minamata. The source of the mercury proved to be the Showa Denko chemical factory forty miles up the Agano River from Niigata. The victims eventually numbered about 500. The outbreak was nicknamed Niigata-Minamata disease. Victims were quick to take the chemical company to court, especially since the company was not part of the community. The people of Niigata were furious. They joined forces with the people of Minamata and inspired them to fight Chisso with renewed vigor.

Finally, twenty-nine families representing forty-five victims of Minamata disease sued Chisso in June of 1969. The trial was long and tedious. One witness, an engineer who had been the head of the Chisso plant at Minamata at the time of the outbreak, was on the witness stand during trial sessions for over a year. He admitted that although Chisso had proclaimed the waste material safe after the installation of the cyclator, he knew that the water was, in fact, not safe. It was apparent from his testimony that company officials felt no moral responsibility for the damage they had done. A company doctor, on his deathbed at the time of the trial, testified that he had told company officials that Chisso was indeed the cause of the illness, but had allowed himself to be silenced by the company.

On March 20, 1973, the verdict was reached. It was the end of an historic and monumental trial, and the plaintiffs were the victors. Their compensation requests were met in full. The Kumamoto District Court decreed:

> . . . It must be said that a chemical plant, in discharging the waste water out of the plant, incurs an obligation to be highly diligent; to confirm safety through researches and studies regarding the presence of dangerous substances mixed in the waste water

as well as their possible effects upon the animal, the plant, and the human body, always availing itself of the highest skill and knowledge; to provide necessary and maximum preventive measures such as immediate suspension of operation if a case should arise where there may be some doubts as to safety. . . . In the final analysis . . . no plant can be permitted to infringe on and run at the sacrifice of the lives and health of the regional residents . . .

The defendant's plant discharged acetaldehyde waste water with negligence at all times, and even though the quality and content of the waste water of the defendant's plant satisfied statutory limitations and administrative standards, and even if the treatment methods it employed were superior to those taken at the work yards of other companies in the same industry, these are not enough to upset the said assumption . . . the defendant cannot escape from the liability of negligence.

Chisso was found guilty and had to pay. The decision awarded $68,000 for deceased or severely ill patients and a minimum of $60,000 for less severe cases, plus a monthly allowance. By early 1975 Chisso had paid indemnities of more than $80 million for its indiscretions against the environment and against mankind. Honest men presided in the courts; the truth became known, and justice prevailed.

In their pictorial essay *Minamata,* W. Eugene Smith and Aileen M. Smith describe the Minamata tragedy and a similar situation involving methyl mercury in Canada. Fish in the English-Wabigoon River in Ontario had accumulated high levels of mercury, and the contamination had been traced to the Dryden Paper Company plant. The pollution affected an area that offered some of the best sports fishing in Canada. In fact, this was a great tourist attraction. The finding of mercury in the fish was covered up and the government made no move to prosecute the company. Dryden did reduce the amount of mercury it dumped into the river to what was considered a "safe" amount, but scientists calculated that the fish would not be fit to eat for many years due to the previous pollution. Concentrations as high as 28 parts per million were reported in the fish. The current maximum allowable concentrations of methyl mercury in the United States is 0.4 ppm. The fish from the English-Wabigoon River pose a hazard especially for the local Indians who subsist on the fish. Sports fishermen carrying home large amounts of fish for the freezer are also at risk. Local people already are exhibiting early symptoms of methyl mercury poisoning.

The Smiths postulate that the reason for inaction on the part of the government is tourism. There are sixteen fly-in tourist camps along the river. The guides are instructed not to say anything about the mercury problem. If it is mentioned by an occasional tourist, the problem is quickly dismissed as "having been blown all out of proportion."

The lessons of history are indeed difficult to learn.

Mercury has been one of the most highly publicized contaminants of the environment. The increasing pollution of rivers and lakes with mercury has halted commercial fishing in some areas, and cases of human and animal poisoning have been reported in addition to the Minamata disaster.

Fish pose the greatest threat of mercury poisoning in the food chain, but birds also have been shown to accumulate mercury, presumably from eating mercury-treated seed used by farmers for planting crops. A Swedish study found high mercury levels in pheasants in a farming area where cereal seed dressed with either methyl mercury dicyaniamide or ethyl mercury chloride was used. No mercury levels were detectable in birds from areas where the mercury-coated seed was not used. It has also been found that mercury is transferred to the eggs of contaminated birds, concentrating in the yolk of the egg.

An interesting and tragic story of methyl mercury poisoning occurred in the United States in 1970. A family in New Mexico who ate pork from a pig it had killed two months earlier developed the symptoms of methyl mercury poisoning. The three children in the family were afflicted, and eventually their ailment was diagnosed. In hindsight the pig appeared healthy when butchered, but other pigs in the herd had signs of muscular uncoordination. For several weeks prior to butchering, the pig, along with the others, had been fed on millet-seed floor sweepings from a local granary. The seed had been treated with methyl mercury.

12
Silver Bay, or Minnesota's Minamata

. . . It must be said that a chemical plant, in discharging the waste water out of the plant, incurs an obligation . . . regarding the presence of dangerous substances mixed in the waste water . . . to provide necessary and maximum preventive measures such as immediate suspension of operation if a case should arise where there be some doubts of safety. . . .

—**Kumamoto District Court**
March 20, 1973

Many a city dweller has daydreamed about leaving the ratrace and traveling to the north woods, where he can no longer see what he is breathing! He envisions a paradise where the air smells fresh and clean, the sky is robin's-egg blue, and the water is cold and pure. He dreams of the silver-white strands of birch reaching to the sky, sandy white beaches, tall pine trees, and sparkling lakes.

Such a paradise is found along the shores of the world's largest fresh-water lake, Lake Superior. There are numerous small towns with low crime rates, where muggings are unheard of and neighbors help each other in times of need. One such town is Silver Bay, Minnesota, with 3,200 inhabitants, eight churches and one bar. Sounds ideal, doesn't it?

But you would probably be much better off living in smoggy downtown Los Angeles. How could this possibly be, you ask? The reason is that the residents of Silver Bay and its neighboring communities have been drinking cancer-causing asbestos in their drinking water for the past decade or more.

Nineteen years ago the Reserve Mining Company, owned by both Armco and Republic Steel Corporations, built a large complex at Silver Bay to extract iron from taconite, a hard black rock found in great quantity in the area. This complex is the nation's largest iron ore processing plant. It produces a significant amount (15 percent) of the country's iron, and in the process produces 67,000 tons of waste rock, or tailings, every day. The tailings are dumped into Lake Superior.

Some historical background of the area is apropos. For years, a red natural ore was mined with open pit mines in the Mesabi range. The ore was rich—about 55 percent iron. It was sent to steel mills without further processing. By the 1950s most of the ore had been mined, and the United States Steel Corporation controlled what was left. Republic and Armco Steel Corporations decided to mine another type of ore—taconite—which is not as rich in iron, containing only about half as much iron as the red ore. Taconite is blasted out of the mine at Babbitt, Minnesota. The ore is crushed and hauled forty-seven miles by rail to the processing plant at Silver Bay, where it goes through a series of grinders and is mixed with water to form a slurry. The slurry is then passed under revolving drums containing electromagnets that attract the iron portion of the ore, which is in turn rolled into pellets and shipped to the steel mills of northern Ohio and Indiana. About two-thirds of the original ore ends up as waste tailings, which are discharged into the bay. There are now five other taconite mines in the area, all disposing of their tailings on land. It was cheaper for Reserve to dump tailings into Lake Superior.

The Silver Bay plant was opened in 1955. At the time it was

considered to be one of the most modern facilities of its kind. Disposal of the waste rock into the lake seemed the best method at the time, and the procedure was approved by both state and federal agencies. If the tailings had been disposed of on land, it would have despoiled the landscape, and returning them to the mine pits would have been expensive.

It was recently discovered that the tailings contain asbestos, the cancer-causing chemical that has resulted in the premature deaths of numerous industrial workers. Most deaths from asbestos have been due to lung cancer, but other deaths have occurred from gastrointestinal cancer, presumably from swallowing asbestos collected in saliva during breathing of asbestos dust, and from mesothelioma, an invariably fatal malignancy of the linings of body cavities that ends by filling the abdomen or chest with tumor.

Local citizens, concerned about their lake, formed the Save Lake Superior Association in 1969. Within two years the association had over three thousand members from Minnesota, Michigan, Wisconsin, and Ontario, Canada. In 1972 one of the members voiced concern that the tailings might contain asbestos. The question inspired the Minnesota Pollution Control Agency to assign a University of Wisconsin geologist, Dr. Stephen Burrell, to study the possibility. Seven months later Burrell reported that there was indeed asbestos in Lake Superior. The Environmental Protection Agency rapidly placed the blame on the tailings from Reserve Mining and advised local residents not to drink water from the lake.

Studies of the drinking water from Lake Superior in towns some distance away from the Reserve plant revealed measurable concentrations of asbestos fibers. A half million fibers per liter of water were found at Beaver Bay, a town southwest of Silver Bay, and even as far away as Marquette, Michigan, asbestos fibers were present in quantities as high as 160,000 fibers per liter of water. Marquette is located about 1,000 miles around the western shoreline from Silver Bay. Even a major city is affected. Duluth, Minnesota, a city of 150,000 located sixty miles from Silver Bay, obtains its drinking water from Lake Superior. Its water contains 20-100 million fine asbestos fibers per liter. After a recent storm the level reached one billion fibers per liter, as measured by the

National Water Quality Laboratory in Duluth. Residents of Duluth have been warned against drinking the unfiltered water.

Dr. Irving Selikoff, professor of enviornmental medicine at Mount Sinai School of Medicine in New York, whose studies helped link asbestos and cancer, said in 1973 that people who continue to drink Lake Superior water "play what amounts to a form of Russian roulette." He pointed out that asbestos has a latency period of from twenty to forty years. Referring to his studies of asbestos insulation workers he said. "After twenty years had passed, their fate became clear. There is no known safe or threshhold level for asbestos.

For the people of Silver Bay the latency period for asbestos has just begun. Reserve Mining has been in operation for only nineteen years, and only since 1965 have large amounts of waste rock containing asbestos been dumped into the lake. It is conceivable that the entire western end of Lake Superior could become a disaster area with an epidemic of cancer in the next ten to twenty years.

Hundreds of families in the area won't drink water drawn from Lake Superior and go to extremes to obtain safe water. When scientists confirmed the presence of asbestos in the water in June 1973, parents were warned by the Environmental Protection Agency not to give young children drinking water from the lake. Many families drove long distances to obtain pure water from springs or wells. Later, water filters became available, and families spent a hundred dollars or more to install filters in their homes. The filters are designed to remove asbestos fibers from the water, but they have the added inconvenience of slowing the flow to a heavy trickle.

Now the Reserve Mining operation is in deep trouble. The asbestos-containing tailings have caused massive pollution of Lake Superior. Furthermore, dust emissions from the operation of the plant also contain asbestos and are polluting the air for miles around Silver Bay.

Like the Chisso Corporation in Japan, the company claims that the tailings are harmless and settle into a small area of the harbor. But even during the 1960s environmentalists and state and federal officials charged that the current was carrying the tailings around Lake Superior, ruining fish habitats and spoiling the beaches.

The final outcome of the Reserve Mining case will be a landmark in the annals of environmental protection. Can a company in the United States of America be closed down or forced to spend millions of dollars to protect the environment in light of public opinion and, more important, in light of new scientific discoveries showing the toxic effects of their pollutants on the human population? So far, this has not been the case. After Reserve Mining decided against a proposed on-land disposal plan, claiming it would cost too much, Federal District Judge Miles Lord of Minneapolis closed the plant on April 20, 1974. It was a courageous decision. But then a three-judge panel of the Eighth U.S. Circuit Court of Appeals reopened the plant a day later. The panel ruled in effect that the government had not made a case for a shutdown because it could not produce a case of cancer caused by the asbestos. This is a dangerous precedent that could weaken antipollution standards. The intention of the standards is to prevent disease before it occurs. It appears that the panel wants a body count before closing a plant.

Economically, the problem is complex. The Reserve Mining facility is going to have to make some costly changes. The company proposed a $187 million project to pump the tailings several miles from Silver Bay into a deep basin created by erecting huge dams of coarse tailings between the surrounding hills. The plan also would include reducing air pollution. However, neither Minnesota officials nor Judge Lord liked the idea. The area involved is adjacent to Palisade Creek, which is prime recreation land, and state officials also point out that a dam failure would allow millions of tons of the asbestos-containing tailings to pour into Lake Superior. The other taconite processing plants in the area discharge the tailings into large, shallow basins several miles across and present no danger to health or the environment. Minnesota state officials want the Reserve tailings dumped near the mining site. This would force Reserve to move its processing equipment from Silver Bay to Babbitt, a distance of almost fifty miles. State-hired consultants said the move would cost slightly over $300 million if all the processing machines are moved. However, Reserve Mining officials said the move would cost considerably more—over $650 million—and the plan is much too costly and could not be justified economically. The company seemed to imply that if it does not get its way it might have to shut down the whole operation.

In September 1974 Assistant Attorney General Wallace Johnson, in charge of the Justice Department's land and natural resources division, asked that the Reserve Mining Company case be settled by the U.S. Supreme Court. He asked that Solicitor General Robert Bork carry the case to the Supreme Court when it began its new term in October. He asked the high court to set aside the ruling by the Eighth U.S. Circuit Court of Appeals to reopen the plant.

Johnson's decision to ask for the Supreme Court appeal was influenced by a letter from Russell W. Peterson, chairman of the Council on Environmental Quality. In the letter he stated:

> Because of the latent effects of carcinogens it will be more than 10 years before the magnitude of the health risk to the people of Duluth and Silver Bay will be fully realized, and unfortunately, it will be based on the fate of 200,000 people. Even a few more days of additional exposure pose an unnecessary and unacceptable risk to the residents of the area. . . .
>
> Reserve undertook to dump waste into the water that created a risk of a health hazard. It now seems equitable to ask that when an enterprise, such as Reserve, undertakes an activity that creates profit for itself and risk of harm to others, and when facts later suggest the possible existence of a health hazard, that it undertakes the burden of proving its activities are safe, rather than force others to prove that its activities are unsafe.

The U.S. Supreme Court refused to hear the case. However, on Friday, March 14, 1975, the Eighth U.S. Circuit Court of Appeals ruled that Reserve Mining Company's discharge into Lake Superior is a risk to public health and must be stopped within a "reasonable" period of time or the plant may be closed. The court refused demands that the nation's largest iron ore processing plant be shut immediately. However, the appellate judges did send the case back to Judge Lord with an authorization to order an end to the plant's hazardous air pollution. The appellate judges indicated that a year was a "reasonable" period for halting the lake disposal of the tailings. The court repeated its earlier finding that becasue no cases of cancer caused by the discharges into the lake had yet been shown, the danger to health was not imminent. The lack of foresight is disturbing. Expert scientists have stated that the situation is extremely hazardous and the reason no cancers have shown up is that the latent period necessary for the disease to manifest itself has not yet passed.

The judges, in ordering a more immediate halt to the air pollution, said that we must recognize that airbourne asbestos is hazardous, even though no cases of lung cancer have yet been attributed to the billions of asbestos particles emitted from the Reserve smokestacks. Why then, have they not recognized the danger of asbestos in the drinking water?

Shortly after the order to cease air pollution, the state of Minnesota and Reserve Mining reached agreement on a $34 million air pollution control program for the taconite processing plant. Believe it or not, the new equipment that is to be installed will capture seven tons of matter each day and discharge the waste material into—you guessed it—Lake Superior! So now Reserve will add seven more tons of taconite tailings to the 67,000 tons it dumps into Lake Superior every day.

There is concern that the appeals court ruling will act as a delaying action. In defining a "reasonable" period of time within which Reserve must stop its discharges into the lake, the court said that this includes time for Minnesota to rule on the on-land disposal site Reserve has proposed or to come up with an acceptable alternative. In addition, Reserve is to be given time to construct the necessary facilities. "We cannot now precisely measure this time," the court declared. If a reasonable period cannot be agreed upon, either party may apply to the district court for a time table.

In early 1976, the Eighth Circuit Court of Appeals disqualified Judge Lord from the Reserve case. The Reserve situation to date is well summarized in the following excerpts from a New York Times editorial dated June 9, 1976, entitled "Judge Lord Was Right":

> "Five months ago a United States Court of Appeals disqualified District Court Judge Miles Lord from taking further part in the case of the Reserve Mining Company because of his alleged

164 / Cancer and Chemicals

"gross bias." The higher court may have had a point about the judge's emotionalism in denouncing the way the company had, in his view, "frustrated the conclusions which had to be arrived at"— but the conclusions themselves continue to be persuasive.

. . . Since Judge Lord's removal from the case, his successor, Judge Edward Devitt, has ordered Reserve to pay some $288,800 for water filtration at Duluth and subsequently fined the company $1 million more for violating water-discharge permits in 1973 and 1974. But he has refrained from ordering the plant to close as long as the company is still negotiating an on-land disposal site for its mining wastes.

Here again the company is obviously in no hurry to move. Late in May [1976] a Minnesota hearing examiner recommended a land site other than the one chosen by Reserve Mining. The company's proposed site would cost it less money but would not, according to the examiner, remove the risk of further contaminating Lake Superior. So the examiner's finding is to be contested.

Reserve Mining . . . has enjoyed the rich profits that come from producing 15 percent of the country's steel manufacture. Its legalistic dodging over a period of *seven years* in order to escape the costs of protecting Lake Superior from the potentially poisonous effects of its operations must be brought to an end.

Should the people in the area develop cancer fifteen years from now as a result of taking in asbestos fibers with their drinking water, they will no more excuse the law's delay than they will forgive the unconscionable reluctance of the Reserve Mining Company to allow considerations of public safety to cut into its profits."

13
Doctoring May Be Hazardous to Your Health

We have the best medical care of any country in the world. The United States had nearly 380,000 physicians, the best medical schools and hospitals. Even with this record, however, our medical care is far from optimal. In fact, at times it is even deadly. According to Dr. Robert C. Derbyshire, an official of the New Mexico Board of Medical Examiners and a crusader for stricter medical discipline, 5 percent of all doctors in the United States are incompetent. Probably many more are of borderline competency because of failure to keep up on the latest findings.

Perhaps the greatest danger to patients, however, is the possibility that certain drugs have long-range toxicity that scientists and drug manufacturers have not yet discovered. This possibility is the best argument yet against the indiscriminate use of drugs.

As mentioned earlier, for example, from 1958 to December 1961 the drug thalidomide was prescribed as a sedative and tranquilizer to expectant mothers in Europe. It was later found that many of the women who took the drug early in pregnancy bore children with major birth defects.

165

In 1969 it was reported that there were 247 children of school age with severe congenital deformities attributable to thalidomide in the United Kingdom alone. It has been estimated that there are as many as 3,000 children in West Germany with birth defects attributable to the drug.

The typical deformity is called phocomelia (seal limbs) and consists of shortened or absent limbs. Associated defects include absence or malformation of the external ear, fusion defects of the eye, and absence of the normal openings of the gastrointestinal tract.

A number of other drugs and chemicals that were once thought to be safe are turning out to cause birth defects. A recent example is the drug lithium carbonate. It is used as an effective treatment for manic-depressive psychiatric disorders. Many patients have had relatively high serum levels of this chemical. A recent study has revealed that therapeutic serum levels in pregnant mice resulted in cleft palates in 16 percent of the offspring when the mothers were given the drug on days six through fifteen of the pregnancy. A second study, in rats, also revealed a high incidence of cleft palates. Eye and external ear defects also were noted. A study is currently in progress to determine the incidence of birth defects among offspring of humans who received the drug lithium carbonate during pregnancy.

Another example is the chemical propylene glycol, used as a vehicle for intravenous medications. One well-known drug using this chemical as a vehicle is the injectable form of Valium. Propylene glycol has been found to produce malformations in chickens, yet the drug is still given to pregnant women. Most physicians not only are ignorant of the latest findings concerning propylene glycol, but they are not even aware that it is present in the injectable form of Valium.

Two commonly used tranquilizers, meprobamate and Librium, were tentatively linked to birth defects in a study performed at the University of California and published in the *New England Journal of Medicine* in December 1974. The researchers, from the School of Public Health at Berkeley, stated that the drugs may cause birth defects if taken during the first forty-two days of pregnancy. This study of more than 19,000 births over several years to women enrolled in the Kaiser-

Permanente Medical Care Program revealed that the rate of severe birth defects among children whose mothers took meprobamate during the first several months of pregnancy was four times higher than among children whose mothers took the drug later in pregnancy. The rate for a similar regimen of Librium was three times higher. The women who took meprobamate early in pregnancy also had deformed children two and one-half times as often as women who took no drugs during pregnancy, and Librium takers had birth defects in their children four times as often as non-drug users. One problem with this study is that the number of women taking these drugs is small, and the results were not statistically significant. The findings must be considered tentative until more patients can be studied.

These examples point out the wisdom of physicians who refrain from prescribing medications for pregnant women unless their lives are in danger. Undoubtedly numerous other drugs will turn out to be detrimental in future studies.

The majority of the blame goes to the Food and Drug Administration because it did not require either adequate testing of these drugs prior to their release or testing of old drugs for possible newly discovered effects. The drug companies also deserve some of the blame because they should take the moral responsibility to check drugs for all possible toxicity prior to releasing them even if the FDA does not require them to do so.

Just as dangerous as the indiscriminate use by physicians of drugs that can cause birth defects is the appalling ease with which doctors prescribe drugs that have never been tested for carcinogenicity. New drugs must now be tested for production of birth defects because of the thalidomide disaster, but they still do not need to be tested for carcinogenicity.

Most doctors are not aware that many drugs have not been adequately tested for long-range side effects. In fact, many doctors are not aware of the *known* side effects of some of the drugs they prescribe. The average busy general practitioner in private practice has two main sources for learning about new drugs. One is the advertisements in the medical journals, complete with a picture of a pretty girl who is ever so grateful to her doctor for making her feel better (the side effects and precautions for the drug are listed in very fine print on another page). The second is the drug salesman. The salesman is given an indoctrination course in the new drug by his company. At the end of this course he is able to extol the virtues of the new drug, and after telling the doctor about it, the salesman offers the doctor a new pen or other gift with the name of the new drug plastered all over it, lest he forget. If asked a reasonably intelligent question about research on the drug, however, the salesman often will not be able to answer.

Several drugs that have been used for many years by the medical profession have recently become suspect as carcinogens. For example, during the past several years, doctors have noticed an increased incidence in a rare type of liver tumor. Although this tumor is benign, it is occasionally fatal due to invasion of the tumor into blood vessels in the liver with massive bleeding. This liver tumor, called a hepatoma, is being found with disturbing frequency in young women. The common factor in almost all cases is that the women have been taking birth control pills.

A study of tumor cases from the Ann Arbor area was published in a 1973 issue of the medical journal *Lancet*. Seven cases were reported in women between the ages of twenty-five and thirty-nine. All had been taking birth control pills for two to seven years.

Until recently, these benign liver tumors were so rare that up to 1944, only sixty-seven cases had been reported in medical literature, and most of these were thought to be secondary to liver cirrhosis. Only four cases of hepatoma were diagnosed at the Mayo Clinic between 1907 and 1954. We are definitely seeing an increase in the incidence of this tumor, and birth control pills are implicated as a major factor in their production. Although the tumors are benign, what is most disturbing is the risk for the future. In animal studies this same type of tumor antedates the development of highly malignant tumors when certain chemical carcinogens are administered to the animals. These benign tumors occurring in young women may be harbingers of a much more serious problem.

Some scientists suspect that the formation of these liver tumors is actually caused by a combination of chemical exposures. If due solely to birth control pills, the increase in tumors should have been noted earlier, because birth control pills have been available since the late 1950s. Women on the "pill" even two years or less have been reported to develop hepatomas. The recent introduction of some other chemical into the environment, acting in combination with the pill, may be the answer.

Another way in which doctors can unwittingly do harm to patients is by ordering unnecessary X-rays. A recent report by Ralph Nadar's Health Research Group stated that unnecessary X-rays cost Americans an estimated $1.4 billion annually and may claim as many as 1,000 lives. The author of the report, Dr. Priscilla W. Laws, associate professor of physics at Dickinson College, stated that 30 percent of the 130 million medical and dental X-rays taken annually cannot be justified. The unneeded X-rays are taken for a number of reasons, including poor judgment on the parts of physicians and their desire to protect themselves from medical malpractice suits.

On the other hand, diagnostic X-rays, when used properly, are life-saving. Often an X-ray can reveal a tumor or other abnormality before severe symptoms occur, and early surgery can increase the patient's chances of survival.

Low-level radiation, including X-rays, increases the possibility of birth defects, genetic mutations, and cancer. We receive more than desirable amounts of radiation in our everyday environment from nuclear weapons tests, color television sets, radium watch dials, and high-altitude airplane flights without taking on the additional load of unnecessary X-rays. Diagnostic and therapeutic X-rays are the largest source of man-made radiation exposure in the United States.

Radiation cannot be seen or felt, and the effects of overexposure may not be manifest for years. Pregnant women, young children, and prospective parents assume the highest risks.

Until the early 1950s almost nothing was known regarding the function of the thymus gland, a gray-colored, lobed structure located in the upper chest, just under the sternum, or breastbone. Doctors thought it was a vestigial organ with no current function. In fact, they thought if the gland was too big, it could cause breathing or other problems. It was even implicated in "crib deaths." So in many large medical centers throughout the country, if a doctor thought a newborn child had breathing problems or a large thymus gland, he recommended radiation to the thymus to "shrink" it. Although it was standard medical practice at the time, there was no scientific basis for this "therapy," but it did shrink the gland. It was eventually discovered that the thymus gland is the backbone of the immune system and is important in our defenses against all sorts of diseases, including cancer.

As you may have guessed by now, a significant number of these thousands of children who had their thymus glands irradiated have developed several types of cancer at a rate much higher than usually found in the general population. The rest of them remain high risks for the rest of their lives. There is no question that these cancers are both radiation-induced and doctor-induced, due to the ignorance of the medical profession some years ago. Individual physicians cannot be blamed. What they did was accepted medical practice at the time.

The University of Michigan Medical Center was one of the institutions that performed thymus gland irradiation. Routine chest X-rays were ordered on most newborn infants at University Hospital and on most children referred to the Medical Center for any reason between 1932 and 1954. Children who appeared to have large thymus glands were referred to the radiation therapy department for treatment. During this time, a total of 958 patients received radiation to the thymic region. The incidence of treatments hit a peak in 1937, when 157 patients were radiated. Of the 958 patients who were treated, 754 were less than one year old and 576 were two months old or younger at the time they were radiated. One hundred seventy-four patients were between one and six years old, and the remainder were seven or older.

A course of treatment consisted of either one, two, or three radiation exposures, the usual interval between treatments being three to seven days. The most common dose, given to 661 patients, was 200 r (roentgens), given once. The largest total dose was 1,000 r divided into three courses over a period of two years. One child received 800 r in four divided doses over a two-week period. In contrast, a diagnostic upper gastrointestinal series X-ray exposes a patient to 2 to 3 r, and the maximum recommended allowance for radiation exposure currently is only 5 r per year.

As early as 1958 radiologists at the University of Michigan Medical Center became concerned about the possibility that thymic radiation might make patients more susceptible to malignancies, and a survey of all patients so treated was performed. The investigators were able to obtain follow-up information on 867 of the 958 patients. The average period of observation was over seventeen and a half years. During this time, 99 (11.4 percent) of the patients had died. Five of the 867 had cancer that had developed subsequent to the radiation treatment. In addition, 13 had developed benign tumors of various types. The five malignant tumors are summarized in Table 2.

Table 2
Summary of Malignancies in Michigan Study

Cancer Type	Age When Irradiated	Dose	Age Cancer Diagnosed
Leukemia	10 d.	200 r	5 yr.
Lymphosarcoma	10 d.	200 r	9 yr.
Thyroid	2 mo.	150 r	9 yr.
Brain (astrocytoma)	9 d.	unknown	8 yr.
Cervix	1 mo.	unknown	22 yr.

Other more recent studies at other institutions indicate that these people are indeed more likely than the general population to develop cancer. The most likely malignancies are cancer of the thyroid gland and leukemia. However, numerous other types also are being reported.

A recent report from Israel tells of a similar tragedy. Doctors there used to treat ringworm of the scalp with radiation therapy. It killed the ringworm, but a number of the treated children have developed cancer of the head and neck, especially in the thyroid gland.

It has been estimated that 20,000 children in the United States and 200,000 children worldwide received radiation treatment for ringworm of the scalp during childhood. A dosimetric study indicated that the dose delivered to different locations of the scalp varied from 450 to 850 rads, with the cranial bone marrow receiving about 400 rads, and the brain doses ranging from 175 rads at the surface to 70 rads at the base. The thyroid gland received about 6 rads.

A recent study from the New York University Institute of Environmental Medicine showed the incidence of tumors of the head and neck including the skin, brain, thyroid gland, and parotid gland were higher in a group of 2,215 persons who had received X-ray therapy for ringworm of the scalp between 1940 and 1959. This was compared with a control group of 1,395 individuals who also had ringworm of the scalp during the same period but received treatment other than radiation for the disease. The radiation-treated group also had a higher incidence of psychiatric disorders than the control group.

Another example: doctors used to use a radioactive material, injected into the veins, to outline the kidneys. The material collected in the kidney and the radiation "drew" a picture of the organs on X-ray film. You guessed it again—a few years later, more cancers.

Although diagnostic X-rays expose a patient to a lot less radiation than radiation therapy, experts in radiation biology recommend as little radiation as possible. It would be foolish to refuse a diagnostic X-ray if one has symptoms that suggest disease, but how many X-rays are ordered either for medical-legal reasons or on patient "demand" with no valid cause? Has your doctor ever asked how much X-radiation you have received in the past prior to subjecting you to another X-ray? The greater your exposure, the greater are your chances of developing cancer at a later date.

In this chapter we have discussed several ways in which your doctor may cause you great harm. Many of these problems could be avoided by reexamining physicians periodically for renewal of medical licenses, and by strict testing of drugs prior to their release for use by the general public.

14
Pollution in the
Operating Room

In man's struggle to survive, perhaps his greatest battle has been against physical pain. A great step in that battle, the discovery of inhalation anesthesia, is one of America's greatest contributions to medicine. It is, in fact, one of America's greatest contributions to mankind. Prior to this great discovery, a surgical procedure was a terrifying and excruciating experience, and the surgeon was hampered by the screams and struggling of his patient. The best surgeon was the one who could operate the fastest.

More than 130 years have passed since the discovery of inhalation anesthesia. Following the discovery of diethyl ether and nitrous oxide as inhalation anesthetics in the 1840's, new anesthetic agents have been discovered and new techniques of administration have been developed. Chloroform was used as early as 1847. Cyclopropane was introduced in 1933. In 1956 halothane, a nonexplosive anesthetic, was introduced. It was soon followed by several additional nonexplosive halogenated hydrocarbons, including methoxyflurane (Penthrane) and enflurane (Ethrane). Ether and cyclopropane are not used much in the United States now because they are explosive. Chloroform has been found to be toxic, and it too has fallen into disrepute. The halogenated hydrocarbons introduced since 1956, together with nitrous oxide, are the most commonly used anesthetics today.

These gases are administered through anesthesia machines that are designed to operate at high gas flow rates. Excess quantities of the gases are allowed to escape into the operating room environment, thus exposing the doctors and nurses to low concentrations of the gases. No one seriously considered the possibility that chronic exposure to these chemicals might be harmful to the operating room personnel.

In October 1968 I began a two-year residency training program in anesthesiology at the University of Michigan Medical Center. Within a few weeks I was administering general anesthesia to patients under the supervision of the staff anesthesiologists. Shortly after learning to administer the anesthetic gases I was able to distinguish among the various anesthetic gases, due to the differences in odors. My wife, who had been trained as a nurse, also was able to distinguish them, and she could tell me what gas I had used each day upon my arrival home each evening. It became a game for us, and we assumed that the odors were clinging to my body and clothes. One night, however, I returned home after using methoxyflurane for a case in the morning and administering spinal anesthetics for the remainder of the day. I showered and washed my hair prior to returning home. The moment I walked in the door, some eight hours after exposure to the anesthetic, my wife told me I had been using methoxyflurane that day and she smelled it on my breath.

It was no longer a game. I realized that the anesthetic gases that I breathed in the operating room were being absorbed and stored in my body and slowly released over a long period of time after I left the operating room. I wondered how long these chemicals stayed in the body and how this might affect the health of operating room personnel. I found this vaguely upsetting.

I recalled having had headaches on several occasions while administering methoxyflurane anesthesia to patients. I also recalled an incident that had taken place several weeks earlier. I was checking the anesthesia machine in preparation for anesthetizing a patient with halothane. In order to determine that the vaporizer was functioning properly, I turned it on and placed the anesthesia mask to my face for a moment to smell the presence of the vapor. At that moment one of my professors came into the room, wrested the mask from my hand, and told me never to do that again. He said that if that had been cyclopropane instead of halothane I might be lying on the floor right now with a fractured skull. I told him that I was aware that several whiffs of cyclopropane could render me unconscious, but this was halothane. The professor replied that some anesthesiologists had become addicted to sniffing halothane and that, in any case, it could be toxic to the liver.

That was the first time I realized that halothane could be toxic. After recalling that incident, the realization that I was absorbing and storing halothane and other anesthetics in my body increased my apprehension about the possible occupational hazards of the field. Until then, I had assumed that no one would have been stupid enough to allow operating room personnel to be chronically exposed to these chemicals without first checking on their disease-producing capabilities. I wondered what long-term effects the chronic exposure to the anesthetic gases had on the health of operating room personnel.

I spent the next several evenings in the medical library searching the literature for previous work on the subject. There was very little. A Russian study in 1967 revealed an unusually high incidence of headaches, fatigue, irritability, nausea, and other vague symptoms among Russian anesthesiologists. The author of that study also noted that of thirty-one pregnancies reported in the survey, eighteen ended in spontaneous abortion, two in premature delivery, and one in a congenital malformation.

In 1968 a study from Northwestern University showed a higher-than-normal death rate from reticuloendothelial and lymphoid malignancies among anesthesiologists. This was found in an inquiry into the cause of death among 441 members of the American Society of Anesthesiologists who died between 1947 and 1966. There was also an inordinately high death rate from suicide among the anesthesiologists.

There was another arguably germane study in the medical literature about that time. A study of the cause of death among chemists revealed that a significantly higher proportion of chemists than of other professional men die of cancer. Nearly half the excess cancer deaths were from malignancies of the pancreas and lymphomas. The relevance, if any, is that both chemists and anesthesiologists are exposed to low concentrations of volatile chemicals and gases in the course of their work.

That was the extent of the literature on the subject at that time. Even so, there were hints of dangerous effects from breathing low concentrations of anesthetic gases while working in the operating room. I knew I was on to something.

I discussed the possibility of harmful effects of the gases with various staff members of the department of anesthesiology. With the exception of moral support from one professor, I received little or no help or encouragement. Many of them thought the entire idea was ridiculous.

Still, I was convinced that there was a problem. I became concerned about my personal safety in the operating room. At the time I was thirty years old and the father of two small children. The thought that I was engaged in a hazardous profession was disturbing. For a few days in December 1968 I seriously considered quitting the anesthesiology training program rather than subject myself to the gases every day. Then I came up with a solution. If I could devise a gas trap to remove the excess gases from the operating room, I could keep the exposure at a minimum. I thought about the problem for a few days and was able to devise a homemade scavenging device that worked quite efficiently. It was made from a child's balloon with a hole punched in the side and fitted over the "pop-off" valve of the anesthesia machine so that all the gases coming out of the valve were trapped in the balloon. The neck of the balloon, or the part into which one blows, was connected by means of tubing and connectors to the wall suction device so that the anesthetic gases were shunted through the tubing into the suction device and out of the operating room entirely. It was simple but very effective. I decided to continue in the program, using my device whenever I administered general anesthesia.

My fellow residents, the anesthesia staff, the surgeons, and the operating room nurses all thought I was slightly deranged. Some were amused; others joked about it; and others were derisive. I usually retorted that anything that smelled as bad as the anesthetic gases couldn't be good for you.

I wanted to study the problem of operating room pollution in detail. The obvious first step was to document the concentrations of the various gases the operating room personnel were breathing during the course of their work and determine how long the gases remained detectable in the breath following termination of exposure.

I quickly found out that I could obtain no assistance from my own department in terms of equipment, personnel, or money. I began searching for collaboration in other departments. I needed a gas chromatograph, expertise in its use, and money for supplies and other equipment. I found it down the street from the hospital at the School of Public Health.

Gwen Ball, a research associate in the environmental research laboratories, took an immediate interest in the problem and recognized the potential risk to operating room personnel. She taught me how to use her gas chromatograph and then helped me design and conduct a series of experiments to determine the concentrations of anesthetic gases in different areas of the operating room and the concentrations of the gases in the breath of both patients and anesthesiologists at different intervals after leaving the operating room. Since I received no time off from my clinical duties for this research, I collected samples during coffee breaks and evenings when I was not on call. Gwen and I came up with some interesting findings. Anesthetic gases were detectable in the breath of patients as long as three weeks after they were anesthetized. Anesthesia personnel had detectable levels up to sixty-four hours after leaving the operating room. These studies had not been performed previously, so Gwen and I were quite pleased when our first paper on the subject was published in *Anesthesiology,* the main journal of the specialty. The paper, entitled "Chronic Exposure to Methoxyflurane: A Possible Occupational Hazard to Anesthesiologists," was published in 1971.

While we were conducting the project, several additional papers were published by other investigators. It turned out that I was not the only one interested in the problem. In 1970 a European study reported a 20 percent spontaneous abortion rate among anesthetists in Denmark. In 1971 a study from Stanford University reported a miscarriage rate of 38 percent among nurse-anesthetists and 30 percent among operating room nurses, contrasted with 10 percent among general duty nurses in California.

At that time there were three small studies showing a high incidence of spontaneous abortion among women working in operating rooms. After several more evenings in the medical library, I learned that chemicals which are embryolethal may also cause birth defects and cancer. In October 1970 I finished the residency training program and accepted a position in the anesthesiology section at the United States Veterans Administration Hospital in Ann Arbor. In June 1971 I became chief of the Anesthesiology Service. As part of the package I received my own gas chromatograph and the technical assistance of Judy Endres.

I decided to perform a survey of the nurse-anesthetists residing in Michigan to explore the incidence of cancer and other health problems among the group. For the survey I enlisted the assistance of Dr. Richard Cornell, professor and chairman of the department of biostatistics at the University of Michigan School of Public Health. In January 1972 we sent the first mailing of questionnaires to the 621 nurse-anesthetists in Michigan. After a second mailing to the nonrespondents and literally hundreds of telephone calls, we had a final response rate of 84.5 percent—a remarkable figure for a survey of this type.

Initial scanning of the questionnaires suggested a large number of positive responses to the questions regarding the incidence of malignancies among the respondents. We compared the incidence of cancer in the Michigan group with age-adjusted statistics from the Connecticut Tumor Registry, one of the most accurate tumor registries in the country. The results were clear: the incidence of cancer among the Michigan nurse-anesthetists was three times the expected rate. Furthermore, several unusual types of tumors occurred among the anesthetists: liver cancer, pancreatic cancer in a relatively young woman, malignant thymoma, leiomyosarcoma, and others. These unusual cancers were suggestive of exposure to a chemical carcinogen. We published our data as a separate paper in *Anesthesiology*.

We later analyzed the data on birth defects among the children of the Michigan nurse-anesthetists and found the incidence to be considerably higher when the women practiced anesthesia during pregnancy as opposed to when they did not. In the same study, exploring the possibility of transplacental carcinogenesis, we found that three maliganancies had occurred in two of the 434 children whose mothers had worked during pregnancy. One had a neuroblastoma (tumor of the nervous system) at birth and later developed thyroid cancer. Another child developed a parotid tumor at age twenty-two. Among the 261 children whose mothers did not work during pregnancy, there was one case of leukemia diagnosed at age three. The figures were not statistically significant, but neither were they reassuring.

While we were completing the analysis of the survey data on cancer, Dr. David Bruce from Northwestern University contacted the Department of Health, Education and Welfare's National Institute for Occupational Safety and Health and aroused NIOSH's interest in the problem of operating room pollution. NIOSH promptly called a meeting to discuss the latest findings of those conducting research in the area. The meeting was organized by Mr. William M. Johnson and Dr. Joseph K. Wagoner of the institute's division of field studies and clinical investigations. The five anesthesiologists in the United States who were researching the problem at that time were invited to the meeting. They were Drs. Ellis Cohen and Charles Whitcher of Stanford, Helmut Cascorbi of Case Western Reserve, David Bruce of Northwestern, and myself. Also present at the meeting were Drs. M. T. Jenkins and E. S. Siker, president and president-elect of the American Society of Anesthesiologists, and representatives of other involved professional groups.

The meeting resulted in the formation of an American Society of Anesthesiologists' ad hoc committee composed of the five scientists who attended the meeting and Dr. Byron Brown, a statistician from Stanford. The committee was chaired by Cohen and was charged to perform a nationwide survey of the members of various professional societies made up of persons who work in operating rooms. The survey was performed with the financial support of NIOSH, and the computer center at Stanford University was used to analyze the data from the 80,000 questionnaires.

In January 1973 the committee sent the first mailing of the detailed questionnaires to the 49,585 members of the American Society of Anesthesiologists, the American Association of Nurse-Anesthetists, and the Associations of Operating Room Nurses and Operating Room Technicians—virtually all the full-time operating room personnel in the United States. At the same time, questionnaires were sent to the 23,911 members of the American Academy of Pediatrics and a randomly selected 10 percent of the membership of the American Nurses Association, all of whom were nonoperating room professionals used as controls.

Several problems were inherent in a study of this type. Certain professional groups had relatively low response rates, and respondent bias was a limiting factor. But in spite of these and other problems, we found reasonable evidence that exposure to the operating room environment entailed a variety of health hazards, particularly for women working in operating rooms and their offspring. The survey revealed that female physician-anesthetists and nurse-anesthetists experienced up to twice the risk of spontaneous abortion of pregnancy as did women not exposed to the operating room environment. Birth defects were twice as likely to occur in the children of nurse-anesthetists as in the children of nurses who did not work in the operating room. There was also a 25 percent increase in the risk of birth defects among children born to the unexposed wives of male physician-anesthetists. This finding was unexpected and somewhat disconcerting, for it suggested that genetic damage could occur in the sperm cells of the exposed males and be transmitted to their offspring. Liver disease was found to occur twice as frequently in anesthesia personnel, both male and female, as in nonexposed groups. Female anesthesia personnel were found to be up to twice as likely to develop cancer as their unexposed counterparts. The data for male operating room personnel were inconclusive.

The results of the study were published in the October 1974 issue of *Anesthesiology*. The committee concluded that there was a significant increase in disease among operating room personnel, and chronic exposure to low concentrations of waste anesthetic gases was the most likely explanation. However, it could be argued that several other aspects of the operating room environ-

ment could exert an influence on the morbidity of personnel—
long hours and tension, for example, and occasional exposure to
radiation from X-rays and radium implantation procedures. A
case could also be made that workers in the operating room are
exposed to patients with a variety of illnesses and that some of
these diseases, including cancer, might be virus-borne and therefore transmissible. However, it would require an extraordinarily
recalcitrant bias not to consider the strong likelihood that a
chemical agent related to anesthesia is responsible for the high
incidence of cancer and birth defects seen especially among the
anesthesia branch of the surgical team.

In the publication of the national survey, the committee
called for further study of the situation and advised women to
avoid working in unscavenged operating rooms during the first
three months of pregnancy. The committee also recommended
that gas-scavenging devices be installed on the anesthesia
machines in every one of the 25,000 operating rooms in the
country.

Anesthesia equipment manufacturers became interested in
producing gas-scavenging devices about the time of the 1971
report from Stanford. The devices first became commercially
available in 1972.

The results of the national survey supported my intuition
that at least one of the anesthetic gases was a carcinogen.
Although the study was not published until October 1974, the
committee members were aware of the findings in late 1973.
Again I began spending all my spare time in the medical library,
this time studying chemical carcinogenesis. I came across an
article describing the carcinogenicity of two halogenated ether
compounds, bis (chloromethyl) ether (BCME) and chloromethyl
methyl ether (CMME). The article had been published in the
Archives of Environmental Health in 1968 by Dr. Benjamin Van
Duuren, director of the laboratory of organic chemistry and
carcinogenesis at the New York University Medical Center. I
immediately noticed the similarity of the structures of the
carcinogenic compounds to several commonly used anesthetic
agents that are also halogenated ethers.

Halogenated ethers constitute a large class of compounds

that have wide use in industry, mostly as intermediates in chemical synthesis. Because they are highly reactive in terms of biologic activity, they had been under investigation by Van Duuren and his staff since 1964. They found both BCME and CMME to be potent carcinogens in mice and predicted that these agents would be found to be carcinogenic in humans and warned that extreme caution should be exercised in their use to avoid skin contact or inhalation. Their warnings went unheeded at that time.

I called Van Duuren in New York, introduced myself, and explained that I was very interested in his studies. I asked whether he was aware that several halogenated ether compounds were being used as inhalation anesthetics. His response was memorable, and I relate the conversation verbatim:

VAN DUUREN: "These anesthetics are not being used in people, are they?"

CORBETT: "Yes."

VAN DUUREN: "Oh, good God!"

I visited Van Duuren the following week. Based on his studies, Van Duuren found one anesthetic—isoflurane (Forane)—particularly suspicious. He thought methoxyflurane and enflurane were also suspicious and should be tested as soon as possible. Isoflurane, fortunately, had not as yet been released by the FDA for use on the general public. It was still an investigational drug, although it had been approved for human clinical trials in seventeen hospitals throughout the country.

Van Duuren also suspected that halothane, the most commonly used potent inhalation anesthetic agent, might be a liver carcinogen. Finally, he predicted that trichloroethylene would be determined to be carcinogenic because of its route of metabolism and its similarity in structure to vinyl chloride.

We concluded that the anesthetics in question must be tested as soon as possible. We agreed to work together; he would advise as I proceeded with the testing. I was a complete novice in carcinogenicity testing. The first step was to begin a pilot study to teach me the techniques and procedures.

Upon my return to Ann Arbor I requested reimbursement for my trip to New York from the University of Michigan

Department of Anesthesia. I was turned down and told that I was embarking on a "wild goose chase."

Several weeks later, Van Duuren visited me in Ann Arbor to discuss the pilot study. We had to limit the study to only one anesthetic agent because of the lack of funds, equipment, and personnel. Our decision on which anesthetic to test first was based on the comparison of their chemical structures with those of chemicals known to be carcinogenic.

The reader may better understand the comparison of chemical structures if we look at a more popular chemical—vinyl chloride. Vinyl chloride has been found to cause a rare form of liver cancer among industrial workers who breathe it in gaseous form during the course of their work. As with most carcinogens, it takes many years for the cancer to develop. The anesthetic agent trichloroethylene has the same basic structure as vinyl chloride, but it has chlorine atoms in place of two hydrogen atoms in the molecule. It is both interesting and frightening that vinyl chloride itself was once considered for use as an anesthetic agent. It does produce anesthesia when breathed in the proper concentrations, but the chemical has an irritant effect on the heart, so it was banned for use as an anesthetic.

Figure 3 shows the similarities among several anesthetic agents and several known human carcinogens. The inhalation anesthetics have never been tested for carcinogenicity. The outlined areas of the first two carcinogens, bis (chloromethyl) ether and chloromethyl methyl ether, are thought to be the portions of the molecules responsible for their carcinogenic effects. The first anesthetic shown, isoflurane, has an identical structure. This relationship prompted us to study isoflurane first.

We also had another reason for studying isoflurane first. If we obtained data suggesting carcinogenicity of this chemical, we could hope to persuade the Food and Drug Administration to withhold its release until more conclusive studies could be performed. We could thereby prevent exposure of millions of patients and thousands of operating room personnel to the chemical.

Carcinogenicity testing of chemicals is very expensive and very time-consuming. We decided to perform the preliminary

Figure 3

Similarities Among Selected Carcinogens and Anesthetics

Human Carcinogens

Inhalation Anesthetics

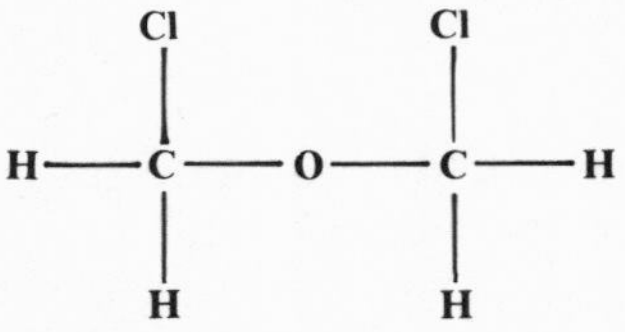

Bis (Chloromethyl) Ether

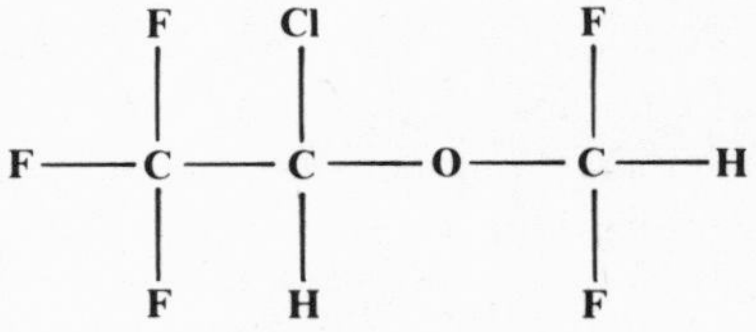

Isoflurane (Forane)

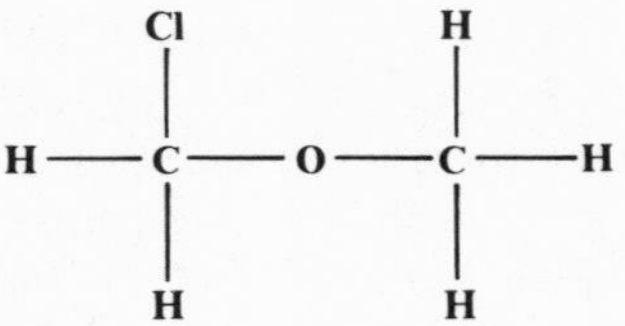

Chloromethyl Methyl Ether

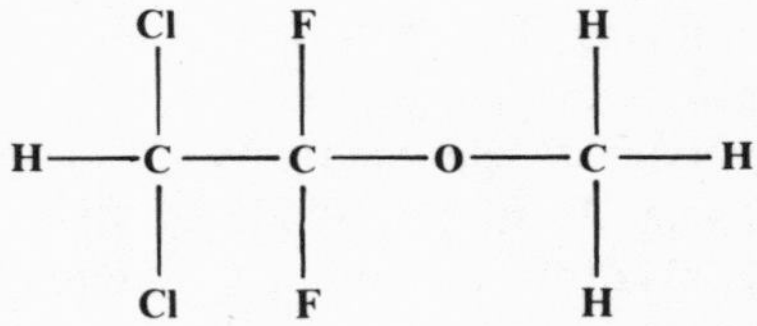

Methoxyflurane (Penthrane)

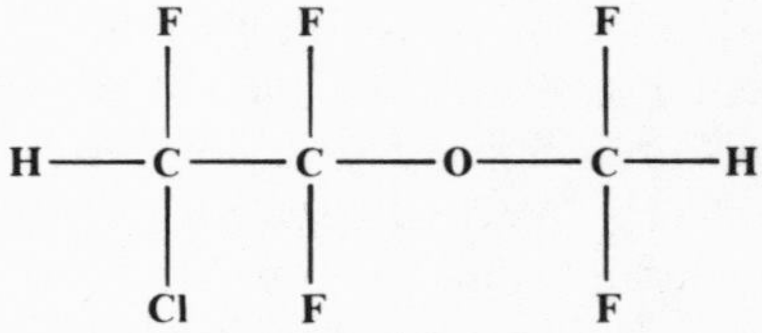

Enflurane (Ethrane)

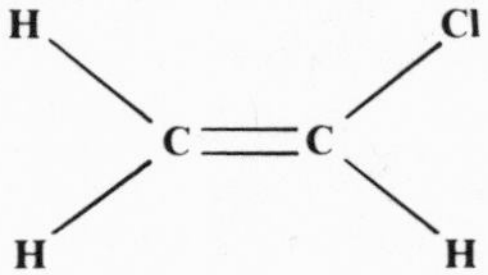

Vinyl Chloride

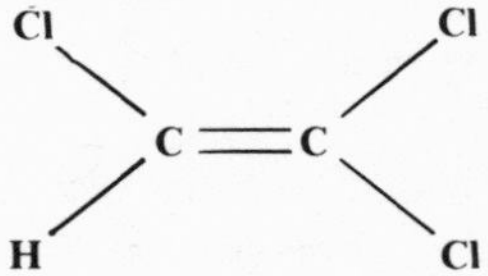

Trichloroethylene

study at the Veterans Administration Hospital in Ann Arbor since I had an exposure chamber there that I was using for other research. The only anesthetic delivery system available could deliver the isoflurane in oxygen, not in compressed air. To further complicate matters, there was not enough exposure chamber time to run an oxygen-exposed control group. As a result, we had to design the preliminary study with several deficiencies. We would not be able to prove beyond the shadow of a doubt that the drug was carcinogenic. However, if the animals did develop tumors after exposure to the anesthetic, we could state that the agent was suspicious and perhaps force full-scale testing prior to its release. This is how we had to proceed.

The next problem was to obtain a few bottles of isoflurane. I called James Vitcha, the product manager of the Ohio Medical Products Company, which manufactures isoflurane under the brand name Forane. He agreed to send a few bottles. I then asked if he knew whether anyone had performed carcinogenicity studies with isoflurane. He said that carcinogenicity studies were not required by the Food and Drug Administration and the company had no plans to conduct or support such studies. I let the subject drop.

After the isoflurane arrived, I ordered animals with some extra VA research funds, and we were off and running. The design of the study was as follows:

Groups of timed-pregnant Swiss/ICR mice were exposed to either 0.5 percent (5,000 ppm) isoflurane on days 12, 14, 16, and 18 of the pregnancy (Group 1) or to 0.1 percent (1,000 ppm) isoflurane on days 12, 14, and 16 of the pregnancy (Group 2). The offspring of both groups were then exposed to 0.1 percent isoflurane every other day from age 5 days until they had received 25 exposures. Each exposure period lasted two hours and was conducted in 8-cubic-foot exposure chambers. The gas mixtures of isoflurane in oxygen were delivered from a Forreger anesthesia machine with a copper kettle vaporizer. A control group of timed-pregnant Swiss/ICR mice and their offspring were exposed to room air only. Groups of offspring were killed and autopsied at ages 3, 6, 9, and 15 months.

We began the experiment in April 1974. We suspected that the three-month examination was much too early to show any carinogenic effect from the drug, but since this was a new type of study for my staff, the experience would be valuable. We did find several benign lung tumors in the experimental animals, but this might be expected since this strain of mouse does occasionally develop this tumor spontaneously.

In October 1974 the animals were six months old. We examined fifty more animals in each group. This time the incidence of lung tumors in the control group was 6 percent while the low-and high-dose groups had 18 percent and 10 percent respectively. This was suggestive, because an increase over the usual spontaneous incidence of tumor in experimental animals is considered a sign of carcinogenic activity.

We performed a nine-month sacrifice of animals in January 1975. This time the findings were more interesting. The lung findings still appeared suspicious, with 5 percent of controls and 15 percent and 28 percent of experimental animals having lung tumors, but the differences still were not statistically significant. The most interesting finding at the nine-month examination, however, was the presence of three liver tumors and a uterine tumor in the experimental animals. None was found in the controls. Liver tumors are not normally found in these mice, especially at such a young age. This was a highly suspicious finding and predicted that more would develop as the animals grew older.

Once I had processed the tissues and confirmed the tumors by microscopic examination, I called Van Duuren to discuss what we should do about our findings. We decided that the manufacturer should be notified. I called Dr. E. I. Eger, II, a research anesthesiologist at the University of California Medical Center at San Francisco, who was an advisor to the manufacturer, and told him of our study and our results.

On February 13, 1975, Eger and two representatives from the company, Vitcha and Dr. Ross Terrell, flew to Ann Arbor to observe and discuss the results of our work. Eger, acting as consultant to the company, questioned me in great detail about every aspect of the project. We discussed the lack of certain control groups, which I had already mentioned to him. At the time he felt the results were meaningful despite the lack of additional controls. We discussed all other possible factors that might make the data invalid. At the end of the afternoon, Eger turned to Vitcha and Terrell and said that in light of the information presented, he thought the drug could not be released at the present time. More studies would have to be performed because these preliminary studies suggested that isoflurane has carcinogenic properties.

On February 20, 1975, Eger wrote a letter to Vitcha stating that in light of their satisfactory review of the experimental design, as well as the equipment and animals used, the results and their implications could not be discounted. He then went on to outline further studies that should be performed, and concluded the letter by writing that:

> . . . if Forane is significantly more carcinogenic and does not evidence any counterbalancing redeeming feature in this [proposed future] study (e.g., lower mortality, less hepatotoxicity) then Dr. Corbett has done mankind (and incidentally, Ohio) a service for which we must be thankful.

Eger, not having a background in chemical carcinogenesis, felt that if *other* anesthetics were found to be carcinogenic, perhaps it would still be all right to use isoflurane (Forane) as an anesthetic. Experts in chemical carcinogenesis feel that *no* agent found to be carcinogenic should be used for anesthesia since alternate drugs and techniques are available.

On February 27, 1975, I visited Dr. Selikoff at the Mt. Sinai Medical Center in New York. We discussed the work I had done with isoflurane and with polybrominated biphenyls. He expressed interest in both problems and offered much help and encouragement. Prior to the visit, I had spoken with Selikoff by telephone concerning our findings and suggested that Selikoff communicate with Eger concerning his impressions of my study. On February 24, 1975, Eger wrote to Selikoff, and on March 13, 1975, following my visit, Selikoff wrote the following letter to Eger:

> Dear Dr. Eger:
>
> Thank you very much indeed for writing me in detail concerning Tom Corbett's studies of Forane. The information was clear, complete and judiciously outlined.
>
> Your comments were obviously correct concerning the

experimental design, including the limited duration at this time, the lack of oxygen stress of the controls and the fact that other anaesthetic agents were not investigated simultaneously. I could add that question might be raised concerning the chemical purity of the test material.

Nevertheless, I share your prudence that, despite these variations, not unexpected in a pilot experiment, the finding of the liver nodules and the uterine neoplasms surely suggests caution at this time. This is especially true since we are now aware of a variety of halogenated hydrocarbons which have been found carcinogenic (carbon tetrachloride, chloroform, vinyl chloride, ethylene dichloride, ethylene dibromide, DDT, PCB's, aldrin, dieldrin, benzene hexachloride), in addition to the active alpha chloroethers as bis-chloromethyl ether.

Many of us, as you, are insecure in evaluating mouse-to-man relationships (I would call your attention to a very thoughtful paper by Marvin Schneiderman and his colleagues of the National Cancer Institute on the subject in the recent Vinyl Chloride Monograph of the New York Academy of Sciences). Perhaps we are coming closer to the possibility of obtaining valid judgments, with the recent demonstration of the predictive value of animal testing by Van Duuren with bis-chloromethyl ether and by Maltoni with vinyl chloride.

Dr. Hans Popper is reviewing the histological sections that Dr. Corbett kindly made available to us.

At first I thought the Ohio Medical Products Company was simply going to accept the knowledge that isoflurane was a suspected carcinogen. Eger, who was an independent advisor to the company, went as far as to say that assuming the findings were valid and the studies were confirmed by repeat experiments, we had made a major contribution to mankind (by preventing exposure of millions of people to a carcinogen), and Ohio Medical Products should be grateful to us for discovering the carcinogenicity of the drug before it was marketed. However, this did not impress the corporate management.

Several weeks later the head of the anesthesia department of a large eastern hospital called and told me that he was contacted by the company and told that Forane would not be coming out as scheduled. This anesthesiologist had performed clinical research on Forane and was lecturing around the country regarding his studies. He told me that he was scheduled to lecture again soon, so the company informed him that there was a new study out that suggested some problems with the drug, but the study was not a very good one. He said the company implied that the drug would be released eventually. This doctor was suspicious of the company's comments, and he had heard "through the grapevine" that I was the "culprit."

Because of our experimental data, the Ohio Medical Products Company canceled a large promotional campaign that had been scheduled in anticipation of final release of Forane by the Food and Drug Administration. The campaign was to have been initiated at the annual meeting of the International Anesthesia Research Society in Hollywood, Florida, in March 1975. On February 17, 1975, I received a call from Dr. T. H. Seldon, the program chairman for the IARS meeting. Seldon requested that I present my data at a special session. Since the promotional program on Forane had been canceled because of my study, he felt the presentation of the data would be a main attraction of the meeting. After discussion, Van Duuren and I decided that we had enough data for a preliminary report, so I agreed to present the material.

During the presentation I stressed that the most important part of the study was its predictive value. The findings were only suggestive, but we had an indication that the experimental animals were going to develop many more tumors as they grew older.

Selikoff discussed my paper at the meeting and compared the halogenated anesthetics with other chemicals that were known to be carcinogenic. He called for full-scale testing of these anesthetics as well as for extensive epidemiological studies of operating room personnel, pointing out that most environmental carcinogens require at least twenty years to produce cancer in humans and that most of the anesthetics currently used have been employed for less time than that.

At the time of the Florida meeting, a spokesman for Ohio Medical Products told the *Wall Street Journal* that the company regarded the results of my study as "very preliminary in nature," and on March 27, 1975, the company sent a letter to hospitals licensed to use the drug for human clinical investigation. The letter called attention to my study "because of misinformation already circulating regarding the implications of Dr. Corbett's work and the significance attached to this very preliminary pilot investigation." The Ohio company letter went on to describe the experiment but omitted the most important finding—the presence of the liver tumors and the uterine malignancy in the experimental animals.

The week following the IARS meeting, I presented a paper on carcinogenicity and teratogenicity of anesthetics at the New York Academy of Sciences Conference on Occupational Carcinogenesis in New York City. I included the results of the Forane study in that presentation. The paper was received with considerable interest by the delegates.

However, when I presented the data at the annual meeting of the Association of University Anesthesiologists in Atlanta several months later, the paper was attacked by at least a dozen anesthesiologists. The attacks were based on points that were either erroneous or irrelevant. The anesthesiologists knew very little about chemical carcinogenesis and carcinogenicity testing.

I tried to point out to the anesthesiologists that the importance of the study was in its predictive value. I stated that this was already becoming manifest. Several more experimental animals had died of malignancies since the data had been presented at the IARS meeting in March.

They still argued. I was asked how I could in good conscience try to prevent the release of a drug with so little data. I was even accused of being a "publicity hound," since the story had been covered by the *Wall Street Journal.* Several of the anesthesiologists present even went so far as to call the editor of the IARS Journal, International Anesthesia Research Society's *Anesthesia/Analgesia Current Researches,* and ask him to withhold publication of the paper. My only defense was to state that time would tell which of us was right.

By June the initial furor over our nine-month data was diminishing, and anesthesiologists were again anxiously awaiting the arrival of isoflurane. It appeared only a matter of time before the drug was released by the FDA. I was in dire need of additional data to support my suspicions.

By this time the mice were fourteen months old. I contacted Dr. Emmanuel Farber, a pathologist at the University of Toronto and one of the foremost experts on mouse liver tumors induced by chemical carcinogens. Farber earlier had expressed interest in our study. He now advised that we perform exploratory abdominal surgery on several mice to see whether more tumors were present. Upon doing so, Judy Endres and I found that two of five experimental mice did indeed have liver tumors. I then decided that it was time to examine the remainder of our animals.

We began examining the rest of the mice in the experiment the second week of July. We were soon aware that we had an ample supply of liver tumors in the experimental mice and none in the controls. It took several weeks to prepare the tissues for microscopic examination and confirmation. Because of the large number of liver tumors in the experimental animals, I again called Eger to notify him of our latest findings. He and Terrell again visited our laboratory, this time on July 21, 1975. During their visit I killed and examined two experimental animals that I had saved for the occasion to demonstrate the procedure to the visitors. One of the animals had no less than five separate liver tumors. Eger performed a statistical analysis of the data. The company official, Terrell, also seemed impressed with the new data.

I told Eger and Terrell that I would not be able to compile the data to send to the Food and Drug Administration for several months because I had other pressing commitments, I wanted the Ohio company to know of the delay so it could plan accordingly.

The company planned accordingly, all right. I thought the company officials would see the handwriting on the wall and stop plans to market Forane. I heard nothing from the company following the visit.

On September 3 one of the members of the anesthesiology department at the University of Michigan Medical Center informed me that a detail man from the Ohio Medical Products Company was telling people that the company expected Forane to be released by the FDA prior to the annual meeting of the American Society of Anesthesiologists in Chicago in mid-October and that the company was planning a big promotional campaign for the drug at the meeting.

Since Eger and Terrell had visited my laboratory and seen the mouse liver tumors in the experimental animals exposed to

Forane, I did not believe that the company would go ahead with its marketing plans. Now I did.

I called Terrell and asked him about the company's plans. He admitted that the company had applied for final FDA approval and expected it in time to promote the sale of Forane at the Chicago meeting.

"Ross," I asked, "how can you in good conscience plan to release that drug? You and Ted have seen the mouse liver tumors!"

He explained that he was not part of the final decision-making process.

"Then," I said, "you had better make it known to those who made the decision that I will be delighted, assuming that future tests prove that Forane is indeed a carcinogen, to serve as an expert witness on behalf of anyone who cares to sue them for a Forane-induced tumor. I shall tell the court that the drug was categorized as "highly suspicious" and they knew this prior to its release. The drug could conceivably be passed by the FDA because I have not yet informed them of the latest results of my preliminary study and because the advisory committee is composed of anesthesiologists who are not knowledgeable about chemical carcinogenesis. However, I have explained the dangers to you and you now know. If the drug later proves to be a carcinogen, which I highly suspect it will, your company won't have any buildings left once the lawsuits are settled."

I was furious. I had the distinct impression that since the company knew of my studies and had later applied for final release of the drug without telling me, it was trying to sneak through the approval before I had a chance to inform the FDA of my latest results.

I had initially thought that we were having a civilized exchange of scientific information. Now I felt that I was dealing with barbarians.

When I called Selikoff to inform him of the situation, he suggested getting expert diagnosis on the tumors from Farber in Toronto. "He's one of the best there is on mouse liver tumors induced by carcinogens," he said. "Ask him to look at the tumors. If he confirms that the drug is dangerous, ask him to write you a letter to that effect and send a copy to the FDA."

The next morning I was on a plane to Toronto with slides in hand. I had called Farber and he had agreed to meet with me, taking time from an already overloaded schedule. He examined the slides while I explained the details and the shortcomings of the preliminary study. Again, I mentioned the critical nature of his evaluation as he finished examining the slides.

"I have to know whether we have enough data here, taking into account the inherent defects in the preliminary nature of the study, to warrant witholding release of the drug."

Farber said yes, the data were ample to consider the drug "highly suspicious," and full carcinogenicity testing must be conducted prior to exposure of humans to the chemical under any circumstances. "I'll back you up all the way," he said.

I returned to Ann Arbor and called Dr. Margaret Clark, acting director of the FDA's division of surgical-dental drug products, to notify her verbally of our findings. I followed the telephone conversation with a complete written report and later sent the report from Farber. I also sent copies to Eger and Terrell.

Meanwhile, Ohio Medical Products was so sure that it was going to get final approval of Forane in time for the American Society of Anesthesiologists meeting that its representatives were continuing to tell anesthesiologists around the country about it and disparaging my study at the same time. I was informed that the company went so far as to have party hats with "Forane" printed on them for anesthesiologists to wear at the meeting.

A week or so prior to the meeting the Ohio company realized that final approval would not be forthcoming in the foreseeable future. Again it had to cancel its promotional campaign.

Clark of the FDA later informed me that she was trying to establish a program of mandatory testing of all anesthetic gases for carcinogenicity, but it was a time-consuming procedure. Meanwhile, the decision on Forane would be held in abeyance while our data were studied by various people within the FDA and by outside consultants.

This is the status of Forane at the present writing. One can only hope that the FDA will decide to withhold release of the drug pending thorough carcinogenicity testing.

This may now indeed by the case because in early 1976, the FDA published in the Federal Register a proposal requiring carcinogenicity testing of all inhalation anesthetic agents.

The Forane story was well documented by Paul Brodeur in the November 24, 1975, issue of *The New Yorker*. The story was received with mixed feelings by people in positions of responsibility within the American Society of Anesthesiologists. On the one hand, I was dropped without explanation from the ASA Committee of Effects of Trace Anesthetics on Health. On the other hand, the article by Brodeur was selected as the first place winner of the 1976 journalism awards program of the society.

15
It's Not Nice
to Fool
Mother Nature

The premise that we might some day "pay the piper" for over-population is certainly not a new one. There are two gentlemen to whom we are indebted for postulating this theory over one hundred years ago. They are Thomas Robert Malthus and Charles Darwin.

Malthus was an English economist and demographer who lived from 1766 to 1834. Malthusian theory states that population tends to increase at a geometrical ratio, while the means of subsistence increase more slowly, at an arithmetical ratio, and this will result in an inadequate supply of the goods supporting life. When the human population exceeds the food supply, nature has three mechanisms for restoring the balance: famine, disease, and war. In 1798 Malthus explained that without these periodic checks the birth rate would so far exceed the death rate that the multiplication of mouths would nullify any increase in the production of food.

Malthus said that the only other alternative to over-population was "sexual restraint." He was an economic pessimist, viewing poverty as man's inescapable lot. He pointed out that issuing relief funds or supplies to the poor encouraged them to reproduce all the more, adding to the problem. Such an attempt at solution would merely postpone the calamity.

In nonindustrial societies Malthusian theory seems to have a potentially threatening validity. Industrial societies, however, have so far refuted the postulations of Malthus. National income has tended to outpace population growth and the size of the family has become a function of choice due to the prevalence and adequacy of the various types of birth control.

It is interesting that it was Malthus who set Charles Darwin on the train of reasoning that led to the theory of natural selection.

Darwin (1809–1882) was an English naturalist who first established the theory of evolution in his monumental work *The Origin of Species.*

From 1831 to 1836 Darwin sailed in *HMS Beagle* as a naturalist for a surveying expedition. His observations of the relationships between geographically separated and time-separated animals led him to reflect on the contemporary prevailing view of the fixity of species.

In October 1838 he read Malthus' *Essay on the Principles of Population.* His own observations had convinced him of the struggle for existence, and upon reading the views of Malthus, it at once struck Darwin "that under these circumstances favorable variations would tend to be preserved, and unfavorable ones to be destroyed. The result of this would be the formation of a new species."

Hence, the theory of natural selection, or "survival of the fittest," was born.

In the nonhuman animal world the *fittest* individuals or groups are those whose physical and behavioral traits make them best able to survive in their environment. This is also true of human animals, yet man is different. Man lives under social and cultural as well as biological rules. His technology, combined with his intelligence, allows him to survive under conditions that would kill him if he were a nonhuman animal. Man's intelligence can be manifest in may forms—the ability to comprehend complex situations and to solve problems; military acumen;

scientific, mathematical, and engineering ingenuity; business acumen, and so on. Intelligence combined with the basic instinct of aggressiveness is an especially "fit" combination for survival in the human situation.

The economists and demographers of today say that Malthus was short-sighted because he could not anticipate Cyrus McCormick and the International Harvester Company, which, along with other companies and modern-day fungicides and insecticides, feed the world.

But we must now consider a possible corollary to the Malthusian theory. Was he possibly right all along? Industrial societies have so far refuted his theory to a great extent, but are we only temporarily prolonging our ultimate fate? Might not the products of our highly industrialized, highly civilized society eventually be the death of us, causing new diseases that will in the end reduce our population to manageable levels, with only the most "fit" surviving? In this case the "fittest" would be those who were smart enough to limit their exposure to noxious chemicals and those with the greatest genetic resistance to their effects.

I suspect that economists and demographers fifty years from now, assuming some of them are left, may look back and say that the short-sighted economists and demographers of today could not anticipate that the very chemicals and machines that fed the world's overpopulation eventually killed all but the most resistant to their effects. They would agree that Malthus was indeed a true prophet and that Darwin's process of natural selection still reigns supreme.

After devoting a lifetime to writing their now classic series, *The History of Civilization,* Will and Ariel Durant wrote one final book summarizing what they had learned from their years of study and writing. This final volume is entitled *The Lessons of History.* In it they state:

> . . . the laws of biology are the fundamental lessons of history. We are subject to the processes and trials of evolution, to the struggle for existence and the struggle of the fittest to survive. If some of us seem to escape the strife or the trials it is because our group protects us; but the group itself must meet the tests of survival.

They also wrote:

> . . . freedom and equality are sworn and everlasting enemies, and
> when one prevails the other dies. Leave men free, and their natural
> inequalities will multiply almost geometrically . . . In the strug-
> gle for existence some individuals are better equipped than others
> to meet the tests for survival. Since Nature has not read very
> carefully the American Declaration of Independence or the
> French Revolutionary Declaration of the Rights of Man, we are
> all born unfree and unequal: subject to our physical and psycho-
> logical heredity, and to the customs and traditions of our
> group. . . .

I suspect that if Malthus and Darwin could be watching
television today, they would enjoy the commercial in which
Mother Nature comes on the screen surrounded by peace and
tranquility. A voice says, "Here, Mother Nature, try some of
this." Mother Nature tastes the product and says, "Why, it's my
sweet, creamy butter!" The voice interrupts, "Fooled you,
Mother Nature! It's new Chiffon margarine!" Mother Nature
raises her arms in anger. Winds howl! Lightning strikes! Mother
Nature unleashes her fury! Malthus and Darwin would nod
knowingly at each other as Mother Nature screams:

"It's not *nice* to fool Mother Nature!"

16
How to Decrease the Risk

Now that we have completed our discussion of the various carcinogens in the environment, the time has come to discuss how you can decrease your chances of getting cancer. This is accomplished by following a few simple rules designed to minimize your exposure to these carcinogens. These rules fall into the following categories: (1) location of residence, (2) diet, (3) personal habits, (4) occupation, (5) consumer products, and (6) medical treatment.

Location of Residence

The first thing to try to avoid is living in the hustle and bustle of a highly industrialized, densely-populated area such as the northeastern United States. This is one of the highest-risk areas. New Jersey is especially noted for producing a variety of different cancers.

A good general rule is: Don't live in a large city with heavy industry. But some smaller towns are not without problems either. For example, the towns in Ohio where vinyl chloride and polyvinyl chloride manufacturing facilities are located, including Painesville, Ashtabula, and Avon Lake, are high-risk areas.

Even certain towns in the wide open spaces are not safe. If you consider moving to the western United States, stay away from Butte or Anaconda, Montana, where the rate of lung cancer is extraordinarily high. And don't be deceived by the beautiful scenery along the western shore of Lake Superior, around Silver Bay and Duluth, Minnesota. There is a high cancer rate there already, and scientists predict that it will rise much higher because of the asbestos in the drinking water.

Unfortunately, it is difficult today to find a low-risk area. If one is seriously considering a move to decrease the cancer risk, the best source available is the National Cancer Institute study mentioned earlier—*Atlas of Cancer Mortality for U.S. Counties: 1950–1969* (DHEW Publication No. 75-780). A study of the incidence maps will reveal safe areas up to 1969. Unfortunately, even this method of selecting a location is not foolproof because of the rapidly changing environments in many locations. What was a safe area several years ago might actually be a high-risk one today. In considering any area that was low-risk in the NCI study, find out whether there have been any new suspected industries or mining operations introduced in the past twenty years. If so, stay away from them—the rates of cancer will be going up!

Diet

Diet is a major factor in decreasing your chances of getting cancer. You can start by not eating processed meats containing sodium nitrite. It is easy to tell which products contain this chemical, because contents have to be listed on the label. Some of the most common sodium nitrite–containing products are hot dogs, bologna, and other luncheon meats, bacon, hams, Spam, corned beef, and similar products.

If you like beef liver, you might be in trouble if the beef has been produced in the United States. Our cattle are given the hormone DES to fatten them. DES is the chemical that causes cancer in young women whose mothers received the hormone during pregnancy, and the liver is the organ that concentrates the hormone the most. Other countries have prohibited the use of DES in livestock.

Next, avoid foods with artificial colors and flavors. Many colorings and flavorings have not been tested adequately for carcinogenicity, and it is likely that at least some of these additives are harmful.

Watch out for peanut butter, and use only the popular brands from large companies. Most larger companies are very strict about detecting the presence of aflatoxins, which can cause liver cancer in very small amounts. Don't buy cheaper, unknown brands, and above all, don't make your own from moldy peanuts!

Personal Habits

There is a lot you can do here. Give up all your vices! Stop smoking and stop drinking. If you are smoking two or more packs of cigarettes a day and drinking yourself into oblivion every night, you're headed for trouble!

If you drink, don't buy cheap brands. They are less refined. However, even the best grades of scotch contain carcinogens in addition to the alcohol. If you smoke a lot *and* drink excessively your chances of getting oral cancers especially increase. If it will help discourage you from smoking and drinking, I might mention that with certain types of oral cancer, the only hope of cure is to have a grossly disfiguring operation, and even then the cancer may well come back and kill you in several years.

If you are young and female, give up sex for a while! Women who get sexually involved with a number of different men before the age of fifteen or sixteen have an increased risk of getting cancer of the cervix at a relatively young age, even in their twenties. While we're on the subject of sex, the next rule is: don't take birth control pills. In addition to the risks of thrombophlebitis (blood clots), heart attacks, and stroke, we can now add liver tumors. The last bit of advice in the category of sex is: if you have spotting or other symptoms, see your doctor right away. If cancer of the cervix is diagnosed early, it is often curable. Don't wait a few months before you go to him. Better yet, get a Pap test at least once a year.

Occupation

Lung cancer is especially high in certain occupations. It can be an extremely unpleasant way to die, and the five-year survival rate is only 15 percent. To decrease the risk, you should refrain from a variety of occupations, including working with asbestos in any capacity. Working with insulation materials, sanding floor tiles, rust-proofing automobiles, and even working as a mechanic with brake linings will make you a sitting duck. You can also get lung cancer by working with the chemical bis (chloromethyl) ether. BCME is found in the textile industry as well as in the chemical industry. You can even get lung cancer by working in steel mills where "coke" is made to fire the furnaces or by working in a smelter in a mining town.

Bladder cancer is an especially rampant disease among certain chemical workers. Unusual kinds of cancers occur with certain chemicals, for example, angiosarcoma of the liver occurs in vinyl chloride workers. You could not pay me enough to work in a vinyl chloride plant, or even live in a town where one is located. Probably the worst job in the plant is that of cleaning the polymerizing tanks after each use. This involves scraping the PVC from the walls of the reactor vessel. The worker breathes high concentrations of vinyl chloride in the process. It may take twenty years to get the cancer, but when it occurs, it is deadly. There is no cure.

You may risk getting leukemia or one of the lymphatic cancers if you work with benzene, which is used as a solvent in a number of products, including glues. You may also risk these diseases if you sniff gasoline regularly. It contains up to 8 percent benzene.

Probably many other occupations increase your chances of getting cancer, but we don't know about them yet. To summarize, stay away from any job or profession that will expose you to a number of different chemicals in high concentrations.

Consumer Products

Since regulatory agencies do not effectively eliminate all toxic substances from consumer products, there are numerous products available that can increase your chances of getting cancer. As consumers, we have a problem in that we do not know which products are dangerous and which are not. If we are exposed to a wide variety of products, sooner or later we will undoubtedly be exposed to a variety of carcinogens.

Vinyl chloride products associated with foods are almost certainly a high risk. Many foods are packaged in polyvinyl chloride containers. Fatty foods and alcoholic beverages packaged in PVC containers collect the highest concentrations of vinyl chloride. Newer manufacturing processes have reduced the amount in polyvinyl chloride considerably. This is a step forward, but exposure to the plasticizers remains the same.

Other food containers also are suspicious. The popular white styrofoam disposable coffee cups contain suspicious chemicals. I recommend not using them until they have been adequately tested. Clear plastic PVC cups are also risky, especially when they are used for alcoholic or hot beverages. Both vinyl chloride and plasticizers will migrate into whatever you are drinking under these circumstances.

Aerosol spray cans also are risky. Stay away from them as much as possible. Avoid breathing deeply when you do use them. Hairsprays and insecticides are especially dangerous. Some older spray cans even contain vinyl chloride as the propellant.

Medical Treatment

Your doctor can do a lot to help you decrease your chances of getting cancer. Do not insist that he prescribe pills for every minor complaint. Most of the pills he is likely to prescribe have not been tested for carcinogenicity. Tranquilizers, powerful analgesic combinations, and hormones are especially suspicious. Insist that he avoid ordering *unnecessary* X-rays (especially for medical-legal purposes), particularly the kind where you get fluoroscoped. Remind him of the carcinogenic risk associated with radiation—the more you are X-rayed, the higher the risk.

There you have it—six categories in which you can help decrease your chances of getting cancer. Unfortunately, some of the steps are rather difficult to follow.

There is one additional step you can take that will benefit not only you, but your countrymen as well. Write your legislators and insist that they enact a tough toxic substances control act.

Practically speaking, it may be impossible for you to avoid all the risks pointed out in this book, but any that you can avoid now will decrease your chances of getting cancer in the future.

Good luck!

Index

205

208 / *Cancer and Chemicals*

Lord, Miles (Federal District
   Judge), 161–64
Lovelock, James E., 77

Magnesium oxide (Nutramaster),
   121–26
Malthus, Thomas Robert,
   195–98
Maltoni, Cesare, 39–41
Mason, Thomas, 99
Meprobamate, 166, 167
Mercury. *See* Methyl mercury
Mesothelioma, 31, 32
Methoxyflurane, 173, 182
Methyl mercury, 148–56
Methylene chloride, 62
Michigan Chemical Corporation,
   121, 137, 139, 140
Michigan Department of
   Agriculture, 125, 135, 136,
   138–40, 142–45
Michigan Department of Natural
   Resources, 110, 137
Michigan Department of Public
   Health, 138, 145
Michigan Farm Bureau Services,
   Inc., 121–26, 136, 137, 139,
   143
Michigan, Lake, 84, 109–10
Michigan Salt Company. *See*
   Michigan Chemical
   Corporation
Milham, Samuel, 50, 51
Milliken, Governor William, 135,
   140, 142
Minamata disease, 147–55
Minnesota Pollution Control
   Agency, 159
Molina, Mario J., 77–79
Monosodium glutamate (MSG),
   62, 63
Monsanto Corporation, 112
Moore, John A., 138
Mycotoxins, 103–5

Nader, Ralph, 34
National Cancer Institute (NCI),
   44, 46, 53, 62, 99–101
National Institute for
   Environmental Health
   Sciences, 138
National Institute for
   Occupational Safety and
   Health (NIOSH), 26, 29, 33,
   37, 46, 49, 179
National Water Quality
   Laboratory, 160
Nelson, Norton, 35
Neoprene. *See* Chloroprene
New York Academy of Sciences
   Conference on Occupational
   Carcinogenesis, 12, 190
Nitrosamines, 55–59
Northwest Industries, 85, 121, 137
Nutramaster. *See* Magnesium
   oxide

Occupational Safety and Health
   Act of 1970, 26
Occupational Safety and Health
   Administration (OSHA), 26,
   37, 41, 80
Ohio Medical Products Company,
   188–89, 191–93
O'Keefe, Patrick, 137–39, 141
Ozone layer, 77–79

Packaging materials, 74–76
Palmer, Alan, 80
Pesticides
   Arsenic, 83
   Bis (2-chloroethyl) ether, 83
   Beta-propriolactone, 83
   Chlordane, 84, 85
   DDT, 81–85
   Dieldrin, 83, 84
   Heptachlor, 84, 85
   Kepone, 52–54, 86
   Lindane, 84, 85